CHIROPRACTIC MANUAL OF
Low Back and Leg Pain

CHIROPRACTIC MANUAL OF
Low Back and Leg Pain

J.E. Thomas, DC, FACO
Diplomate in Orthopedics, 1973
Fellow of the Academy of
Orthopedics, 1983

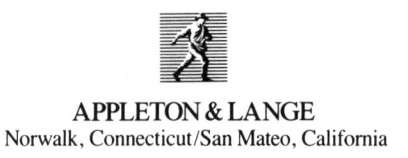

APPLETON & LANGE
Norwalk, Connecticut/San Mateo, California

0-8385-1096-5

Notice: Our knowledge in clinical sciences is constantly changing. As new information becomes available, changes in treatment and in the use of drugs become necessary. The author and the publisher of this volume have taken care to make certain that the doses of drugs an schedules of treatment are correct and compatible with the standards generally accepted at the time of publication. The reader is advised to consult carefully the instruction and information material included in the package insert of each drug or therapeutic agent before administration. This advice is especially important when using new or infrequently used drugs.

Copyright © 1991 by J.E. Thomas
Published by Appleton & Lange
A Publishing Division of Prentice Hall

All rights reserved. This book, or any parts thereof, may not be used or reproduced in any manner without written permission. For information, address Appleton & Lange, 25 Van Zant Street, East Norwalk, Connecticut 06855.

91 92 93 94 95 / 10 9 8 7 6 5 4 3 2 1

Prentice Hall International (UK) Limited, *London*
Prentice Hall of Australia Pty. Limited, *Sydney*
Prentice Hall Canada, Inc., *Toronto*
Prentice Hall Hispanoamericana, S.A., *Mexico*
Prentice Hall of India Private Limited, *New Delhi*
Prentice Hall of Japan, Inc., *Tokyo*
Simon & Schuster Asia Pte. Ltd., *Singapore*
Editora Prentice Hall do Brasil Ltda., *Rio de Janeiro*
Prentice Hall, *Englewood Cliffs, New Jersey*

Library of Congress Cataloging-in-Publication Data

Thomas, J.E. (James Enos)
    Chiropractic manual of low back and leg pain / J.E. Thomas.
        p.   cm.
    Includes bibliographical references.
    ISBN-0-8385-1096-5
    1. Backache—Chiropractic treatment. 2. Spine—Diseases–
Chiropractic treatment.   I. Title.
    [DNLM: 1. Backache—diagnosis.   2. Backache—therapy.
3. Chiropractic.   4. Pain—diagnosis.   5. Pain—therapy. WE 755
T458c]
PZ265. S64748   1991
617.5' 64 - dc20
DLC   91-4582
for Library of Congress   CIP

Acquisitions Editor: Stephany S. Scott
Production Editor: James Gormley
Designer: Michael J. Kelly

PRINTED IN THE UNITED STATES OF AMERICA

*I dedicate this book to my wife, Marilyn,
and to all individuals who suffer with spinal lesions
that cause pain*

Contents

Foreword xi
Preface xiii
Acknowledgments xv
About the Author xvii

1. Body Regions & Pain Syndromes of Low Back/Leg Pain 1

Introduction 1

Research project for low back/leg pain 1

Pain syndromes 2
    Body regions 2

Pain area identification 3

Low back region 4
    Paraspinal syndrome 4
    Lumbar syndrome 5

Pelvic region 5
    Inguinal syndrome 5
    Gluteal syndrome 5
    Thomas syndrome 6

Leg region 6
    Anterior femoral syndrome 6
    Lateral femoral syndrome 7
    Posterior femoral syndrome 7

Conclusion 7

References 7

2. Anatomy of the Spine 9

Anatomy of the spine related to low back, pelvic, and leg pain syndromes ... 9
    Anatomy of the spinal joint or motor unit 9
    Posterior primary rami 12
    Anterior primary rami 12
    Lumbar plexus nerves 12
    Sacral plexus nerves 13

References 13

3. Nerves to Low Back, Pelvis, and Legs 15

Dermatome versus cutaneous pain areas 15

Nerve and nerve groups and their spinal level 15
    Reactive tissue resulting from neural response 16
    Posterior primary rami 17
    Anterior primary rami 18
    Nerve supply to each syndrome 20

References 20

4. Spinal Lesions 21

Spinal lesions causing low back, pelvic, and leg pain syndromes 21

Definition of a lesion 22
    Definition of a subluxation/disrelation lesion 22

Classification of the spinal lesion 22
    Secondary versus primary spinal lesion 23
    Subclassification of a subluxation/disrelation lesion . 24

Symptoms of a spinal lesion 24
    Response from the posterior primary rami 24
    Response from the anterior primary rami 25

Known symptoms of a subluxation/
disrelation lesion **26**

**Basic information for differential
diagnosis**..**26**

References..**29**

**5. The Mechanism of Low Back/Leg
Pain** **31**

**Recorded findings for low back/leg
pain cases** **31**
    Pain mechanism 32

Conclusion...**34**

References..**34**

**6. Regional Orthopedic Examination
for Low Back/Leg Pain** **35**

Examination procedures **35**
    Straight leg raising (SLR) test 36
    Pain to the back of the leg................37
    Pain at the lumbosacral joint 37
    Pain to back areas other than
    the lumbosacral joint.........................38
    Fabere test 38
    Soto Hall test—Linder's sign............39
    Conclusion of supine position 39
    Sitting—straight leg raising
    (SSRL)...39

References..**40**

7. Spinal Segmental Examination **41**

Vertebral testing................................**41**
    Body position for a segmental
    examination 41
    Examination for spinal segmental
    reaction 41
    Segmental findings............................42
    Conclusion of the prone position......43

**Conclusion for physical examination
of low back/leg pain** **43**
    Segmental examination form............44

References..**44**

8. Paraspinal Pain Syndrome **45**

Paraspinal pain syndrome **45**

Common areas of pain found in this
syndrome...45
Nerve supply to this syndrome
area..47
Characteristics 47

**Examination finding for the paraspinal
pain syndrome** **48**
    Examples...48
    Discussion related to treatment 49

References..**50**

9. Lumbar Pain Syndrome **51**

Lumbar pain syndrome **51**
    Area of pain found in this
    syndrome...52
    Nerve supply to this syndrome
    area..52
    Characteristics 52
    Examination findings for the lumbar
    pain syndrome..................................53
    Examples...54
    Differential diagnosis from the sacroiliac
    lesion...55

Discussion related to treatment........**55**

References..**56**

10. Inguinal Pain Syndrome **57**

Inguinal pain syndrome **57**
    Common areas of pain found in this
    syndrome...57
    Nerve supply to this syndrome
    area..58
    Characteristics 58
    Examination findings for the inguinal
    pain syndrome..................................59

Discussion related to treatment........**59**

References..**60**

11. Thomas Pain Syndrome....................**61**

Thomas pain syndrome **61**
    Common areas of pain found in this
    syndrome...61
    Nerve supply for this syndrome
    area..61
    Characteristics 62
    Examination findings for the Thomas
    pain syndrome..................................63

Discussion related to treatment........**63**

References..**64**

12. Gluteal Pain Syndrome 65

Gluteal pain syndrome 65
   Area of pain found in this syndrome 65
   Nerve supply to this syndrome area 65
   Characteristics 66
   Examination findings for the gluteal pain syndrome 66

Discussion related to treatment 66

References 67

13. Anterior Femoral Pain Syndrome 69

Anterior femoral pain syndrome 69
   Areas of pain found in this syndrome 69
   Nerve supply in this syndrome area 69
   Characteristics 70
   Examination findings for the anterior femoral pain syndrome 71

Discussion related to treatment 71

References 71

14. Lateral Femoral Pain Syndrome 73

Lateral femoral pain syndrome 73
   Area of pain found in this syndrome 73
   Nerve supply to this syndrome area 73
   Characteristics 74
   Examination findings for the lateral femoral syndrome 74

Discussion related to treatment 74

References 75

15. Posterior Femoral Pain Syndrome 77

Posterior femoral pain syndrome 77
   Areas of pain found in this syndrome 77
   Nerve supply to this syndrome area 78
   Characteristics 78
   Examination findings for the posterior femoral syndrome 79

Discussion related to treatment 81

References 82

16. Composite Pain Syndromes 83

Composite pain syndromes 83
   Examples of composite pain syndromes 88

17. Disability Impairment Evaluation for Low Back/Leg Pain 91

Procedures presently accepted by the AMA Guide 91
   Anatomical structures 93
   Determination of pain syndromes 93
   Physical examination 93
   Other examination procedures 93

Discussion related to impairment rating 95
   Rating an impaired spinal joint 97
   Rating an impaired posterior primary rami 98
   Rating an impaired anterior primary rami 98

References 100

18. Evaluation of Treatment for Low Back/Leg Pain 101

   Torsion roll for the thoracolumbar region 103
   Torsion roll for the 4th or 5th lumbar vertebra 104

19. Database on Low Back, Pelvic, and Leg Pain 107

Single pain syndrome cases 107

Double pain syndromes 112

Three or more pain syndromes 113

Totals for the 8 primary syndromes 113

Totals for composite syndromes 114

Totals for all syndromes 115

**Appendix A:
Bibliography for Low Back, Pelvic, and Leg Pain** 117

    Spinal joint lesion 117

    Spinal lesions and pathology (nerves) 118

    Correlation between pain area, spinal nerve, and lesion....................119

    General references 121

**Appendix B:
Recommended Information, Graphs, and Forms for Third Parties** 123

    Types of subluxations 124
    Symptoms of a subluxation 124
    Pain syndromes caused by a subluxation/disrelation injury..................124
    Nerve divisions and major nerves that may be involved in a subluxation/disrelation injury.................125

Forms 101 through 108 127

References for Forms 101 through 108 135

Forms 109 through 112 136

References for Forms 109 through 112 141

Index 143

Foreword

This book about the diagnosis and treatment of back pain may well be one of the most valuable books you will ever read.

As all doctors who treat pathologic conditions of the low back, pelvis, and leg know, by far the greatest percentage of this kind of pain is a result of the stresses and strains of daily living: lifting too much weight, or lifting from an awkward and/or unbalanced posture, twisting oneself into a pretzel while dancing or engaging in sports, falling, being struck, exercising strenuously without the proper warm-up, and many other activities that put undue stress upon the skeletal system.

These kinds of injuries are rarely severe enough to require the extended use of pain-killing drugs or surgical procedures, but they do cause much pain and suffering to their victims.

The problem has always been the isolation of the precise source of the pain. A diagnosis of "low back pain" is the one most commonly given, but is not very specific.

Through his observations of symptoms, the treatment given, and the results of such treatments for hundreds of patients in his office practice, through painstaking record-keeping and the compiling of statistics for these cases, and through reading and organizing all the literature available on the subject of back pain, Dr. Thomas has produced three significant contributions toward a better understanding of, and thus more effective treatment of pain from these debilitating conditions.

He developed a spinal segmental examination procedure that will locate with pin-point accuracy the spinal level causing a patient's pain. (Examination findings are supported most of the time by electroneuromyography (EMG). Although EMG scanning was not done with the patients in the original study for this book, Dr. Thomas has used it with many patients since that time; the high correlation shown between EMG readings and spinal segmental examination findings give objective proof of the validity of this examination procedure).

He classified all low back, pelvic, and leg pain caused by spinal lesions into eight major pain syndromes, and showed that all pain that is caused by a spinal lesion fits into one of these categories.

The first person to ever accomplish this, Dr. Thomas linked the body area of the patient's pain with the nerve or nerves that supply that body area, and also with the spinal level where the root of that nerve or nerves exit from the spinal column. When you think of it, this three-way linkage—from pain area, through nerve pathways, to nerve root—is much more logical than following dermatome patterns that prove to be inaccurate much of the time. It is amazing that it has not been considered before.

Dr. Thomas's book was written primarily to share his research findings with other chiropractors, but would certainly be a worthwhile addition to the library of every professional concerned with health care.

E.W. Balkwell, MS, MEd
Northport, Florida

Preface

The research in, and the statistical compilation of, pain areas caused by spinal lesions has not been considered a glamorous endeavor, and thus has led to an indifference of approach by researchers and physicians. Many authors and physicians have estimated that low back/leg pain affects as much as 80% of the population at one time or another in their lives. One might wonder, then, why a condition as prevalent as low back/leg pain is lowest in the scientific priorities required for its investigation—probably because it is not life-threatening. It is, however, one of the most expensive and debilitating conditions on a national level. It has been stated that there are approximately 20 physicians in the world, both chiropractic and medical, who are conducting research along these lines. Just consider the number of projects and the amount of money spent on other conditions that exist in far less frequency; then consider the public demand for, and the willingness to support, these programs financially. Is it not ironic that no one is concerned about low back/leg pain until it manifests itself?

Doctors who treat this condition must do so without the benefit of a viable diagnostic examination procedure, as no procedure for the diagnosis of low back/leg pain has been approved by the healing arts. Without this diagnostic procedure, findings are inconsistent, with the treatment being based on those findings. This inconsistency is not confined to the diagnosis and treatment of these cases, but, through various reports, extends to attorneys, other physicians, the insurance industry, and third parties. This disseminated inconsistency creates problems in impairment factors that make it difficult to evaluate disability levels equitably. The effect this has on the patient cannot be gauged.

Because the most prevalent symptom is a subjective symptom, pain, researchers in low back/leg pain have been reluctant to use this symptom as a basis for their research. No other single symptom is consistently found, however. True, the symptoms from spinal lesions may be found at many areas, encompassing almost half the body, but how can the researcher hope to understand this complex condition without some knowledge of the pain characteristics? The research that has been conducted for spinal lesions is certainly necessary, and has contributed much information about these lesions, but unless the pain characteristics are known the two factors cannot be joined.

There are many books written by both medical and chiropractic physicians concerning low back and leg pain. Absent from most of those discussions is the link that connects spinal lesions with that pain and the neural system that might be injured, or reactive, and causing pain. Those references which do give some information that these connections exist are forgotten by the healing arts shortly after publication—so, little further investigation proceeds along those lines.

Nevertheless, as early as 1959, one researcher did indicate that injection at the base of the first lumbar spinous process produced pain at the iliac crest. It was further found that injections in the interspinous ligament at the first lumbar caused pain at the iliac crest, the groin, and the scrotum. Pain below the iliac, the groin, and the scrotum was caused by injections at the second lumbar. Pain at the anterior thigh was produced by injection at the third lumbar. Upon injection of the fourth lumbar, pain was produced at the lateral and posterior thigh and the medial ankle. The area covered with pain from injections at the fifth lumbar was the same as that of the fourth lumbar but included the lateral leg.[1] There is recent informaton along the same lines of inquiry published by Finneson. The point is that a greater knowledge and definition of the pain areas arising from separate spinal levels or nerves seems to be the key to the clarification of the mechanism of pain, even though the separation of specific pain areas as been overlooked and neglected until now. The following paragraphs

---

[1] Turek SL. Referred pain from the back. In: *Orthopaedics*. Philadelphia: JB Lippincott; 1959:746.

delineate the present lack of knowledge in this field and also my directions for revising the older corpus of knowledge in these areas.

In *The Chiropractic Journal,*[2] an article was written by Stephen M. Perle, DC, CCSP, stating, "Most practicing chiropractors have seen patients who have pain that does not fit the usual dermatome patterns we were all taught. Accordingly, we were told that dermatome charts are only guides and that variation is common."

My research in low back/leg pain, shown in this text, corrects this lack of knowledge by describing pain syndrome areas that are constant regardless of the type of spinal lesion present; the syndromes differ only in the number of pain areas that might be present and in the severity of the pain.

All doctors who treat pain areas caused by spinal lesions are aware that the pain can be caused by constitutional diseases of bone, birth defects, congenital conditions, changes in spinal kinesiology, and, of course, by spinal joint damage due to injury. There must be some connection between pain caused by osteoarthritis, tropism, spinal curvatures, and injuries to the spine, when the condition is not grossly pathologic, such as in a dislocation. Why is it possible for some patients, who have severe degenerative or traumatic arthritis—even compression fractures, as is often found in osteoporosis—suffer little or no pain, when a seemingly minor injury in other patients, with or without any existing joint pathology, causes severe pain, and often disability? There is the possibility that a potential disc lesion is produced by a relatively minor injury, yet a true disc lesion, in this manner, is so insignificant statistically that it cannot account for the millions of low back/leg pain cases. A disrelation of normal or pathologic joints, especially when it is quick and unsuspected, can disrupt the present function of that joint, both anatomically and neurologically, causing pain.

Every chiropractor has had patients with back pain associated with spinal constitutional lesions, and following a few treatments by specific manipulation, the pain disappeared. There surely was no major change in the constitutional disease, but something was changed. I have treated many children who have injured their backs while playing, and have seen these children grow up, become athletes, or enter the armed services with no further back problems. Some of these individuals, 25 to 30 years later, still do not have a back problem. I am not suggesting that a few treatments of manipulation are responsible for the absence of further back problems, but I am suggesting that back problems do not necessarily stem from childhood injuries unless the injury was not corrected and over a period of many years produced slow degenerative changes. Spinal changes can occur to the adult as well as the child when injured spinal tissue becomes a chronic secondary lesion. When it is possible to correct the lesion found in children or adults, degenerative changes may be aborted.

The spinal subluxation/disrelation lesion is the only spinal lesion that can exist undetected, possibly for many years, low grade and concurrent with a gross pathologic condition, again for long periods of time, and yet remain dormant until a future accident or tissue change precipitates a reaction. It is a condition less than grossly pathologic.

It is time that all members of the healing arts as a whole accept and recognize the existence of the generic subluxation/disrelation lesion, begin to understand its complications, and be aware that physical examination procedures for gross pathology can no longer be accepted as criteria for the physical evidence produced by this lesion. They must be aware that this lesion may exist independently, or may coexist with any other pathologic condition affecting motor units of the spine. Pain syndromes produced by injury or spinal pathology less than an intervertebral joint dislocation are caused by the presence of the subluxation lesion. Precise diagnostic procedures are now available for the detection of an active subluxation, and the ability to rate the reactions of this lesion are a part of that procedure. This knowledge gives the physician a new working tool.

---

[2]Perle SM. Scleretogenous pain defies easy diagnosis. *The Chiropractic Journal* 3(3):20, 1988.

Acknowledgments

Many factors led to the research and desire to write this manual. The first, and to me most important, was the different diagnoses given by several physicians, both medical and chiropractic, for a severe spinal injury my wife sustained. It was at that time that I started recording pain areas suffered by patients, similar to the present method, and began investigating the reasons spinal physical examination procedures and x-ray findings differ so radically from one physician to another. My work during those earlier years was conducted to increase my personal knowledge of spinal injuries and their ramifications, without thought of publication. The encouragement for publication of my material came from Dr. Larry Green of Michigan when he stated that my work should be put in print, that my findings were too important to be shelved when I retire.

The writing and compiling of a desk manual for low back/leg pain is an arduous undertaking that requires help and moral support. My secretary, Deboral Parker, has been a great help. While conducting her normal duties in a daily office practice, she has sorted, arranged, typed, printed, recorded, and given moral support. The artist was Joanne De Boer of Port Charlotte, Florida. David Oaks, a practicing attorney in Punta Gorda, Florida has been helpful in portions of Appendix B. Betty Balkwell, a retired teacher, has spent many hours proofreading this manual; she also wrote the Foreword. David Hughes, manager, and the staff at Computerland have kept my equipment in top condition and have also given much needed advice.

Last, but not least, the Florida Chiropractic Association—its Executive Vice President, Dr. Edward Williams, and staff has played a major role in the evolution of this manual for, by publishing my papers on the subject of low back, pelvic, and leg pain, the FCA thereby helped lay the groundwork of research necessary for this undertaking.

J.E. Thomas, DC, FACO
Port Charlotte, Florida

About the Author

Dr. Thomas has been in private practice since 1949. For the past 19 years, he has conducted clinical investigation in the procedures used for the diagnosis and examination of low back, hip, groin, and leg pain. He is a member of the American Chiropractic Association, the Council on Chiropractic Orthopedists, the Academy of Chiropractic Orthopedists, the Florida Chiropractic Association, and the Florida Council of Orthopedics. He has been a Diplomate in the field of Orthopedics since 1973 and attained a Fellowship in 1983 from the Academy of Orthopedics.

He is past President of the Michigan Orthopedic Society, was Chairman of the Michigan Peer Review Board. He wrote questions on diagnosis for the State Licensing Board and lectured as a member of the National College Teaching Team in the postgraduate orthopedic division. The subjects he taught were Differential Diagnosis of the Spine, Kinesiology, Disability Evaluation, Constitutional Disease of Bone, and Body and Extremity Casting. He is listed in *Who's Who in the Midwest* (15th edition, 1976–1977) as author of a booklet, *Instructions for Constructing Removable Body Casts,* designed for the treatment of certain spinal lesions. He is also listed in *International Who's Who in Medicine* (1st ed. 1987) for his continued work in the diagnosis and examination of low back/leg pain cases.

In 1974, he received the Certificate of Merit from the Michigan State Chiropractic Association for professional services rendered. He received the award for "Clinical Journalism," the highest given by the Florida Chiropractic Association, in October 1986. His most recent award was given him by the Charlotte County Chiropractic Society on March 27, 1987.

Dr. Thomas is the first physician, either chiropractic or medical, to classify and chart low back/leg pain syndromes and their lesions. He also developed a regional and spinal segmental examination procedure, that better enables all doctors to determine the nerves and spinal level involved with an injury or lesion.

His charting of the major low back/leg pain syndromes with statistical information has been a clinical breakthrough. He has maintained a close watch on all forms of treatment related to spinal pain syndromes. He plans to continue his investigation of these problems and to create improvements when possible in the best interest of those patients who suffer pain from spinal injury or disease.

CHIROPRACTIC MANUAL OF
Low Back and Leg Pain

Chapter 1

Body Regions & Pain Syndromes of Low Back/Leg Pain

INTRODUCTION

Low back/leg pain is a highly complex problem that is discussed and written about as if it is a single entity. Terms as shown below are common descriptions given to this condition.

1. Acute and chronic low back pain
2. Acute and chronic low back/leg pain
3. Acute and chronic uncomplicated low back and/or leg pain
4. Acute and chronic complicated low back and/or leg pain
5. Low back strain/sprain

Treatment is often based upon these classifications, with little or no additional differentiation.

It is common knowledge that the use of diagnostic tests such as the x-ray, ultrasound scan, computer assisted tomography (CAT) scan, and magnetic resonance imaging (MRI) are unable to give an effective differential diagnosis for many of these cases. Even the various regional examinations now used for low back and leg pain are inadequate for an effective differential diagnosis.

Because of the inefficiency in the examination procedures, and the void in understanding the causes and classifications of low back/leg pain, I began my research program. This book is based upon that work, which began in the mid 1960s and continues today. The statistics are taken from 572 cases prior to writing this manual. This creates a better understanding that all pain in low back and/or leg pain cases, due to spinal joint lesions, is located in one or more of eight different anatomical body areas, and each one of the eight is supplied by a single nerve, or nerve group for that body area. These nerves or groups, with their spinal level of origin, can be differentiated by first precisely isolating the single pain areas suffered by each case. Those cases with multiple pain areas have either greater damage, or reaction to the single joint, or the involvement of more than one joint with its nerve or nerve group.

RESEARCH PROJECT FOR LOW BACK/LEG PAIN

The original project was to find and record the pain areas suffered by the patient, and to determine their perimeters and location, **regardless of the type of underlying pathology.** This procedure was soon followed by the recording of spinal segments that were painful to percussion and/or probing, again **without regard to the existence of underlying pathology,** and whether or not there was any apparent relationship to the pain area.

By early 1970, I found (1) that the pain suffered by the patient, when carefully charted, did fall within certain defined areas, which turned out to be similar to the cutaneous divisions as described in Gray's and other anatomy texts; and (2) that there were only eight major pain areas found that can be classified as individual "pain syndromes." The fact that pain did not fall into dermatome patterns as we have been taught, and as shown in various texts, was a puzzle that I had to solve. This required an additional 10 years to investigate and understand.

The importance of these major pain syndrome areas must not be underestimated. **All pain caused by spinal lesions exists within one or more of these syndrome areas, and each area is supplied by an individual nerve or nerve group that can be recognized and charted. The spinal root levels from these nerves or nerve groups are well known. We can now, finally, connect pain, nerve, and the spinal lesion into an abnormal unit.**

During this time, the nerve supply to the areas of pain had to be determined and understood. The spinal root level of those nerves had to be investigated and evaluated. The interlinking of both the anterior and posterior primary rami had to be studied. Various regional orthopedic examination tests for low back/leg pain were individually reviewed, with positive and negative findings related to the area of pain studied, and evaluated. It was found that **pain syndrome areas** do not differ among patients having a reactive grossly pathological joint from those cases having an injury to a previously normal healthy joint, providing the joint level, nerve, and/or nerve group is the same. It was also determined during that period that certain orthopedic tests were of greater value than others when properly done and precisely evaluated. These regional tests of most value were then utilized as the basic test for the examination of all cases that suffered from low back and/or leg pain. Because of its extreme importance, the procedures required to determine the reactive spinal segment also became part of that basic procedure. Found only by the spinal segmental examination, the joint reaction is unique in that it can be accurately rated, and that it is directly related to the pain suffered by the patient. Its presence indicates that a subluxation/disrelation lesion exists. The type of lesion may be only the disrelation, or it can be complicated by various forms of gross pathology.

The examination of individual joints of the spine has been a part of chiropractic scrutiny since its beginning; unfortunately, this examination procedure has not been standardized, accorded enough significance, nor has it been refined until now. I believe that the main reason for the neglect our profession has shown this important procedure is because the chiropractor tends to jump to a conclusion based upon the patient's recital of symptoms instead of the actual hands-on examination. He has, therefore, discarded one of the finest tools for the determination of spinal joint reaction the healing arts have known.

The examination of each spinal segment that could be a potential cause of low back, pelvic, or leg pain was improved upon and refined until a specific procedure was developed. Reactive spinal segments were shown to be present following injury to both normal and abnormal spinal joints. Negative reaction was found to be present over normal uninjured joints, and mild reaction to negative findings are found over abnormal joints, dormant or nonreactive joints, not associated with pain syndromes.

The next step in this project was to see if the orthopedic examination findings, the segmental examination findings, the reactive nerve, or nerve groups were related to the pain syndrome areas as suffered by the patient. A definite relationship was established.

Finally, the question to be answered was, would treatment to those reactive segments have a direct beneficial effect in reducing or controlling pain suffered by the patient? In the final step came the most rewarding results of the entire research project. It was found that treatment to reactive segments, determined by the segmental examination, had a direct and beneficial effect in reducing and/or controlling low back/leg pain.

The following chapters will provide the procedures and information in their correct order required for the differential diagnosis of low back/leg pain and will offer a better understanding of the mechanism of low back, pelvic, and leg pain caused by spinal lesions.

PAIN SYNDROMES

A great deal of information is now known or available regarding spinal pathology, arthritis, spondylosis, facet injury, birth defects, curvatures, spinal fractures, and disc lesions, but little of this information has aided in the differential diagnosis and treatment of pain to the low back, pelvis, and legs.[1]

In order to effectively diagnose, examine, and treat the patient who suffers from pain caused by spinal injury or reaction, a precise and orderly examination procedure is necessary. A procedure for low back/leg pain cases, acceptable to the healing arts, had not been available in the past because there were too many unknown factors. Much of the information previously absent is now known, and this knowledge creates a database for low back/leg pain cases. This basic information enables the physician to proceed in all phases of this field, confident that each step is accurate, and that the treatment provided is built upon a solid foundation.

The first step in the diagnosis of low back/leg pain is to isolate the primary symptom suffered by the patient, which is pain, and place it in its proper body region and pain syndrome area. This gives us an accurate location of the pain, and this knowledge aids in the determination of the nerve or nerve group involved supplying that body area. Knowledge of the nerve or nerve group to that body area enables the doctor to locate the nerve root and its spinal level(s).

Body Regions

To pursue the goal of classifying pain areas, we must first divide low back/leg pain areas into three separate regions: the low back, pelvis, and leg. Some basis of identification must be used for this separation. Anatomical landmarks have been combined with known neurological levels as points of division for these regions. Traditionally, pain to the lower body has been classified as low back pain, or low back/leg pain, which is incorrect because it does not indicate the pelvis, an important body area containing nerves subject to pain.

The primary motions of the spine are flexion, extension, side bending, and rotation. The nerve supply for these motions at the lower thoracic region is the dorsal primary division of the spinal nerves;[2] the uppermost anatomical nerve part of this plexus is the 12th thoracic nerve.[3] This nerve is the highest member of the lumbar plexus that innervates muscles of the low back, and is partially responsible for low back motion. Branches from the 9th, 10th, and 11th thoracic nerves also aid in this motion.[4]

Because the 12th thoracic nerve is the highest anatomical nerve of the lumbar plexus and a primary nerve in low back motion, it makes an excellent point to consider as an upper perimeter for the low back pain region. The 12th thoracic vertebra lies between the 11th and 12th thoracic nerves, becoming an anatomical landmark as well as a neurological boundary for the upper perimeter of the low back pain region. The lateral body centerline divides the front of the body from the back. Dorsal nerves follow a downward route.[5] By drawing a line from the 12th thoracic vertebra to the iliac midline of the body, our angle will follow these nerve routes. We now have an apex, the 12th thoracic vertebra, and two sides, the lines drawn from the 12th thoracic to the lateral crest of the ilium.

The base line, which creates a triangle, runs an anatomical course using the lumbosacral junction and the iliac crest as the lower border of the low back region (Fig. 1–1).[6] This region now has both neurological and anatomical bases for its existence. This base perimeter becomes a dividing line between the low back and pelvic region.[7]

The pelvic perimeters are described as follows. The upper border is now the iliac crests connected by the lumbosacral junction. The lateral borders end at the body lateral midline, and the inferior border is bounded by a line along the gluteal fold curving up to the trochanter of the femur.

The greater trochanter of the femur is designated as part of the lower division line because one pelvic pain area extends as far down as the trochanter, and the nerve supply to that pain syndrome is the anterior primary division of the 12th thoracic nerve.[8] This division line from the trochanters to the apex of the sacrum is now the lower border of the pelvis and the only border required for the leg region. Three pain regions are now classified to give an accurate body location for the pain syndromes. Not only do we have a visual location of the pain regions, but this knowledge also gives an indication of the nerve or neural system found within that region, associated with the pain suffered by the patient.

PAIN AREA IDENTIFICATION

The next step is to get an accurate location of the pain from the patient. This may seem like an insurmountable task, but with the following procedure it can be done. Be aware that obtaining the precise pain area creates the foundation that you will be working with. Have the patient with pain at the low back, pelvis, or legs indicate the total area of pain. If the total area covers more than one region start at the low back region and work downward until the patient has outlined all areas of pain within each region. Do not allow the patient to hurry or unintentionally mislead you as to the precise perimeters of the pain. Sketch or shade the indicated areas for each region on a drawing of the body before continuing to the next region. Posterior and anterior drawings are a must. Lateral views may give additional perspective. These drawings with the shaded pain areas will now become a permanent record to be used in all correspondence with third parties. It not only provides an accurate location of the pain area, but a visual outline as well. This record cannot be changed or distorted by a third party for any reason. Used with your progress report, it is invaluable. **(The determination of the pain area, based upon information received from the patient, and its recording, must be done only by the physician.)**

1. Low Back Region
2. Pelvic Region
3. Leg Region

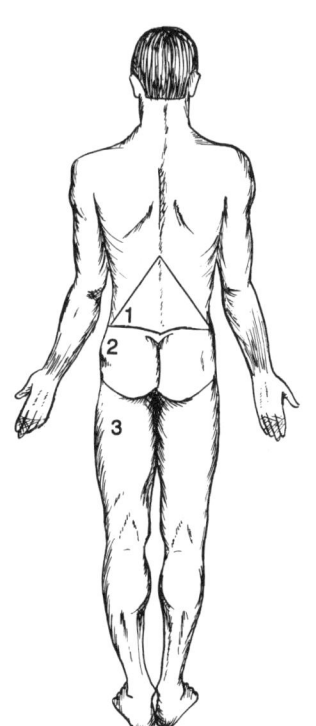

Figure 1–1

Important: The pain syndrome area is a predetermined and constant area of the body supplied by a known nerve or nerve group. The perimeters of this area are not subject to change.

The pain area indicated by the patient is that localized area found within the syndrome area. There may be one or more pain areas found in the syndrome area. These pain areas must be determined before any attempt is made to examine the patient. Once determined and recorded, they are also not changed, even if pain is caused from the examination or the probing of associated tissues. Changes of pain areas within the syndrome area, resulting from treatment, do not change the original recording.

Gather this information in your office at the same time the patient's history and general information are obtained. The examination is conducted later.

As a direct result of the previous procedure, coupled with the regional classification, eight major pain syndrome areas have been found and charted; two in the low back, three in the pelvis, and three in the leg region.[9] Three or four minor pain syndrome areas have been found, but they are insignificant for overall statistics. These are discussed later.

To confirm these eight major pain areas as pain syndromes, criteria for major pain syndromes had to be developed. This is of great importance. Pain not associated with spinal injuries, and transitional pain such as pain caused by contusions, tumors, individual muscle sprain, and so on, should not be recorded as major spinal pain syndromes, even if found within the spinal pain syndrome area. This prevents inaccurate recording of the major pain syndromes.[10] The criteria are as follows:

1. A pain syndrome must exist as a separate area.
2. It must appear often enough to have a statistical basis.
3. It must have a shape that is predictable.

(To clarify the first criterion, there are patients who have two or more pain syndromes, but each major syndrome exists alone.)

LOW BACK REGION

Seventy percent of all single pain syndrome cases are found within this region. They are the paraspinal and lumbar syndromes.

Paraspinal Syndrome

This syndrome is the most common, and it is found in 48% of all low back, pelvic, and leg pain cases (see Fig. 1–2). In single syndromes it accounts for 42%. When the low back region is the only region

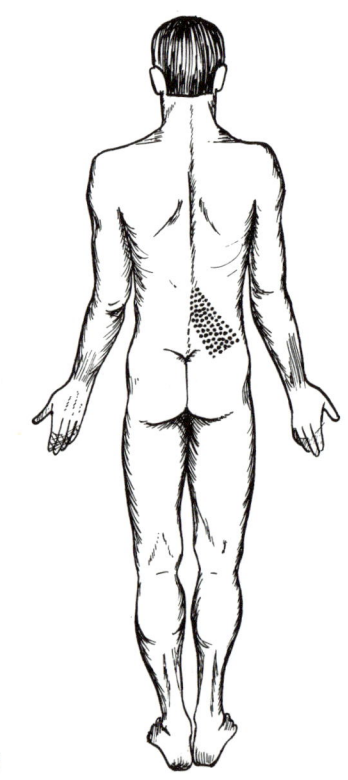

Figure 1–2

involved with pain, the paraspinal and lumbar syndromes are found together in 3% of all cases. The paraspinal syndrome may be present on either or both sides, but it is most commonly found unilaterally. Except for a spot the size of a baseball over the 5th lumbar, all pain from the 12th thoracic to the lumbosacral joint, following the iliac crest to the lateral body midline and angling back to the 12th thoracic vertebra, is covered by this syndrome. It may extend 1 or 2 inches below the iliac crest. If the pain is more than 1½ inches lateral to the 5th lumbar spine, a paraspinal syndrome is present (see Fig. 1–2).

The most common description and area outlined by the patient is unilateral and along the iliac crest. If bilateral, it will be indicated that it hurts entirely across the low back. Should it be described in this fashion, ask if there is pain at the center of the back and indicate the area, if necessary. A paraspinal syndrome is present when a negative answer is given. An affirmative reply assures you a lumbar syndrome is probable. Another common area is lateral to the 5th lumbar at the top of the sacroiliac joint. The patient may indicate small areas anywhere along the crest of the ilium, some radiating obliquely upward. Other patients may have pain radiating downward from the level of the 12th thoracic vertebra. Any pain in the paraspinal pain area should be considered a paraspinal pain syndrome unless proven otherwise.

Lumbar Syndrome

This area of pain is located over the 5th lumbar vertebra and lumbosacral joint. It is approximately 2 to 2½ inches in diameter (see Fig. 1–3). It is found in 28% of all single pain syndrome cases and in 27% of all combined low back, pelvic, and leg pain cases. This syndrome has a dual characteristic.

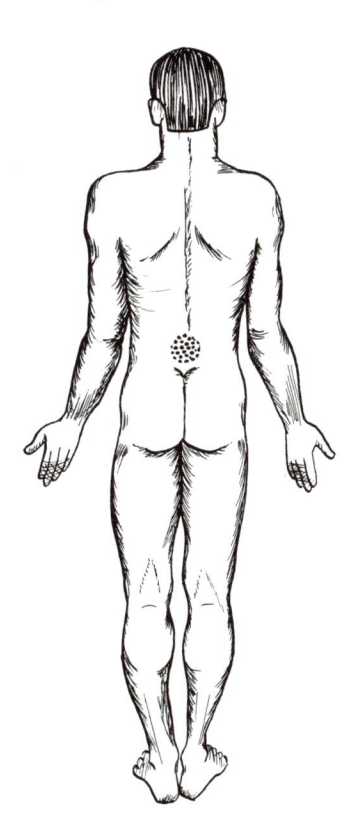

Figure 1–3

It is caused by injury or reaction to the lumbosacral joint, or it may result from injury or reaction found at the supraspinal ligament, with no pain or injury to the 5th lumbar nerve root, motor unit, or disc. Occasionally, both may be present. An incorrect diagnosis here can lead to improper treatment and failure or unsatisfactory results.

PELVIC REGION

Ten percent of all single pain syndromes are found within this region. They are the inguinal, gluteal, and Thomas pain syndromes.

Inguinal Syndrome

It is found in 4% of all single pain syndromes. This syndrome is not a low back pain problem; it is, however, a nerve syndrome arising from irritation or injury to spinal nerves and, therefore, is properly placed as a member of low back/leg pain spinal syndromes. It is divided into two parts. The first and highest portion is about 2 or 3 inches wide, running parallel to the groin and above it. The second and lower is over the groin, extending from the anterior iliac crest to the pubis. The sharpest area is frequently about half way between these two points. This syndrome is often diagnosed as an internal problem, especially in female cases (see Fig. 1–4).

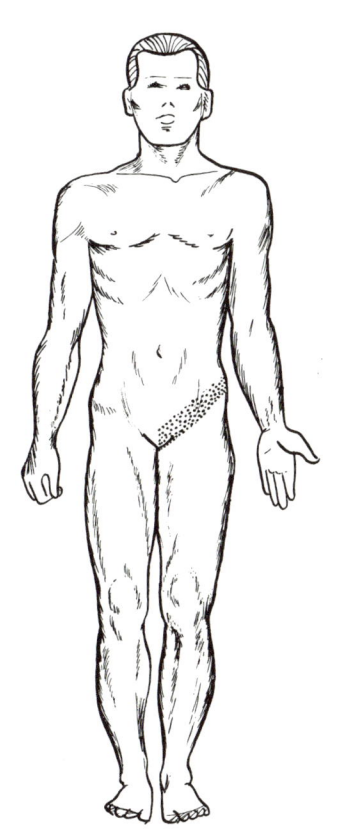

Figure 1–4

Gluteal Syndrome

This syndrome appears in 3% of all single pain syndrome cases. Although not commonly found alone, it meets the criteria for pain syndromes, and must be considered. This syndrome is about the size of a baseball and is located above and lateral to the ischial tuberosity. It is generally persistent and quite painful. Sitting is most difficult when this syndrome is present (see Fig. 1–5).

ful portion is a small triangle that is above the greater trochanter of the femur. It extends upward where the base is approximately 2-inches wide at the iliac crest. The second part extends immediately behind the first portion and fans out over the posterolateral gluteus. If you open your hand and place the thumb at the iliac crest center line, fanning out the fingers slightly, you will fairly well cover this second area of pain (see Fig. 1–6).

LEG REGION

Twenty percent of all single pain syndromes are found within this region. They are the anterior, lateral, and posterior femoral pain syndromes.

Anterior Femoral Syndrome

It is found in 7% of all single pain cases. This pain area covers the anterior portion of the thigh, extending from approximately two inches below the inguinal ligament to the knee. It does not encompass the medial or lateral thigh, but often extends to the medial side of the knee joint. In a small percent of cases, the greatest area of pain is found at the knee. Should this be the case, a careful examination of the knee, possibly including x-rays, might be wise to eliminate any knee pathology (see Fig. 1–7).

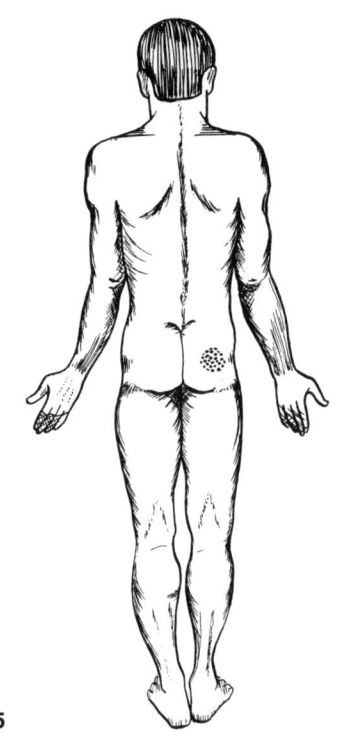

Figure 1–5

Thomas Syndrome

This syndrome is found in 4% of all single pain cases. It was catalogued by the author in 1974. Although it overlays the hip, calling it a hip syndrome would be misleading. It appears in two parts and either or both may be present. The most pain-

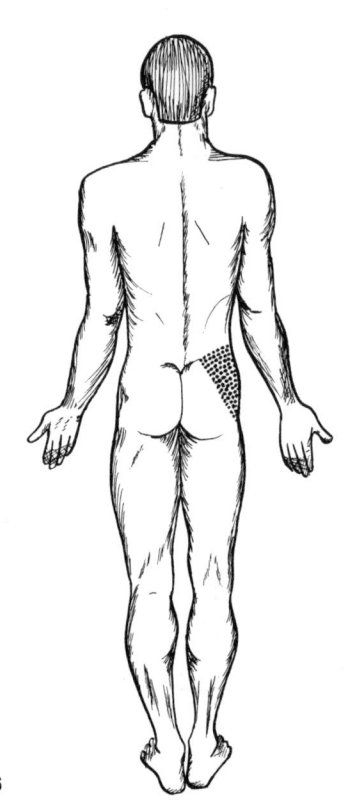

Figure 1–6

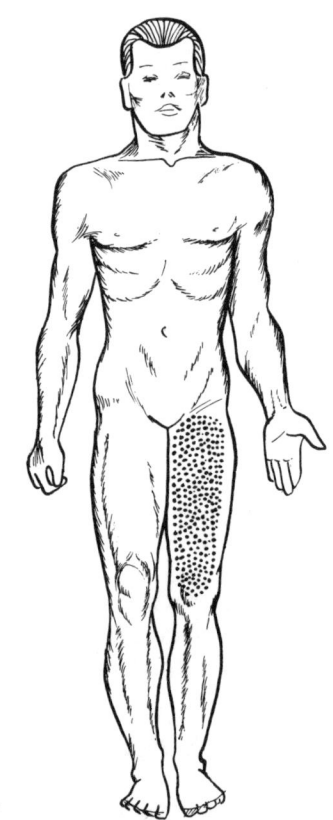

Figure 1–7

Lateral Femoral Syndrome

This syndrome is also found in 7% of all single pain cases. It covers an area from the hip to the knee on the lateral side of the thigh. There are a few cases in which the patient will state that pain is present on the side of the leg, but also extends toward the front of the leg. A lateral femoral syndrome is still the classification. If both the front and lateral areas are covered by pain, a composite is present. Occasionally, the pain will cover only the upper half of the lateral femoral syndrome area (see Fig. 1-8).

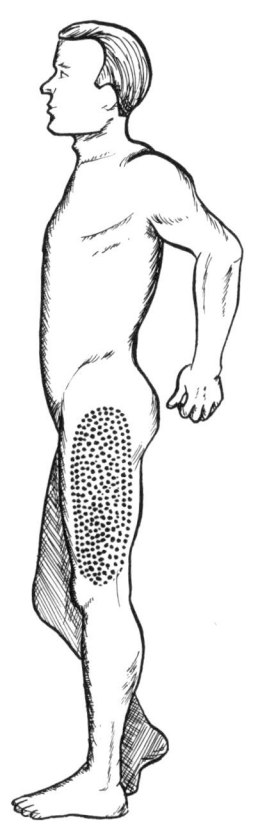

Figure 1-8

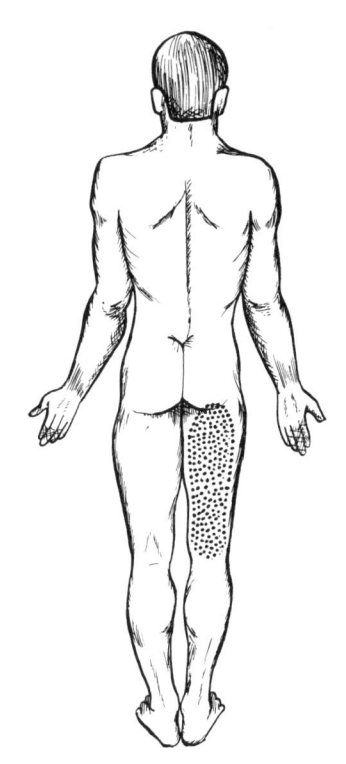

Figure 1-9

Posterior Femoral Syndrome

This syndrome is found in only 6% of all single pain syndrome cases. The area covered by this syndrome is the back of the thigh (see Fig. 1-9). It extends from the lower gluteal region to the back of the knee. Rarely, pain will extend down the posterolateral area of the lower leg to the little toe. This syndrome is most commonly, but mistakenly, diagnosed as a sciatic syndrome caused by a disc lesion.

CONCLUSION

No longer need the broad term *low back, or low back/leg pain* be used. The use of this generic term denotes pain in all these regions. It is not precise enough for a description that must, at times, be used in insurance and legal circles. The chiropractor now has the necessary information to identify regional and specific pain syndromes that isolate the pain area involved, so that an accurate description can be given and understood by all. By charting these pain areas, we find that only eight major pain syndromes exist within the three regions. We also know that these pain syndrome areas are a constant. They can be recorded for a permanent medical history, can be used for information in a progress report, or transferred to another physician or interested party without loss in the translation. They are an effective picture of the patient's pain.

REFERENCES

1. Douglas C, Mooney V, Crane P: Discussion: Pathology not predictive of treatment outcome for low back pain. *Spine* 9(1):94, 1984
2. Gray H: *Gray's Anatomy,* 30th ed. Philadelphia, Lea & Febiger, 1984;p.1193
3. Gray H: *Gray's Anatomy,* 30th ed. Philadelphia, Lea & Febiger, 1984;p.1226
4. Gray H: *Gray's Anatomy,* 30th ed. Philadelphia, Lea & Febiger, 1984;p.1221
5. Gray H: *Gray's Anatomy,* 30th ed. Philadelphia, Lea & Febiger, 1984;p.1197

6. Gray H: *Gray's Anatomy,* 30th ed. Philadelphia, Lea & Febiger, 1984;p.467
7. Thomas JE: Classification of low back/leg pain. *FCA Journal* September–October:39, 1985
8. Gray H: *Gray's Anatomy,* 30th ed. Philadelphia, Lea & Febiger, 1984;p.1223
9. Thomas JE: Classification of low back/leg pain, Part 2. *FCA Journal* November–December:18, 1985
10. Thomas JE: Criteria for major pain syndromes. *FCA Journal* September–October:39, 1985

Chapter 2

Anatomy of the Spine

ANATOMY OF THE SPINE RELATED TO LOW BACK, PELVIC, AND LEG PAIN SYNDROMES

In considering the anatomical structures of the low back, the primary concerns are joints, muscles, ligaments, soft tissue, and nerves, and their relationship to the pain syndromes found in low back/leg pain cases.

The portion of the nervous system most involved in low back, pelvic, and leg pain arises from each vertebral foramen extending from the 10th thoracic level to the lumbosacral joint. This is the area to be reviewed.

There are three thoracic vertebrae, the 10th, 11th, and 12th, and five lumbar vertebrae, the 1st, 2nd, 3rd, 4th, and 5th. The 5th lumbar joint, or motor unit, includes the sacrum. Muscles, fascia, ligaments, and other soft tissue that connect the spine and body trunk to the pelvis are included.

As a unit, the motions of the spine are flexion, extension, lateral flexion, and rotation. The five lumbar segments are able to move primarily in flexion and extension, whereas the thoracic vertebrae move in rotation and lateral flexion. The motions described are allowed or restricted due to the anatomical characteristics of those segments within the given areas.

Each vertebral unit contributes to these motions in varying degrees, depending upon its location in the spinal column. These units do not function alone, but as a member of the group. This factor has caused great difficulty in isolating a spinal lesion without gross characteristics in a diagnostic work-up. These vertebral units of motion are called motor units, and each unit contains individual muscle groups and attachments that enable isolated antalgic muscle contraction for that unit, even though the unit works within the whole.

Anatomy of the Spinal Joint or Motor Unit

This bony connection at the spine can be described in three sections (see Fig. 2–1).[1]

The anterior section contains the body of the vertebra. This body is the primary spinal supporting structure. The disc, or fibrocartilage, lies between two vertebrae, acting as an important shock absorber. The anterior and posterior longitudinal ligaments cover the front and back of this column, respectively.

The middle section contains an opening between the lamina of the vertebra above and below—the *foramen*. It is also bounded in front by the disc, portions of the vertebral bodies, and the posterior longitudinal ligament. The posterior boundary is the ligamentum flavum, articular facets, and the posterior area of the lamina, which are connected to form the posterior spinous process.

The posterior section includes the spinous pro-

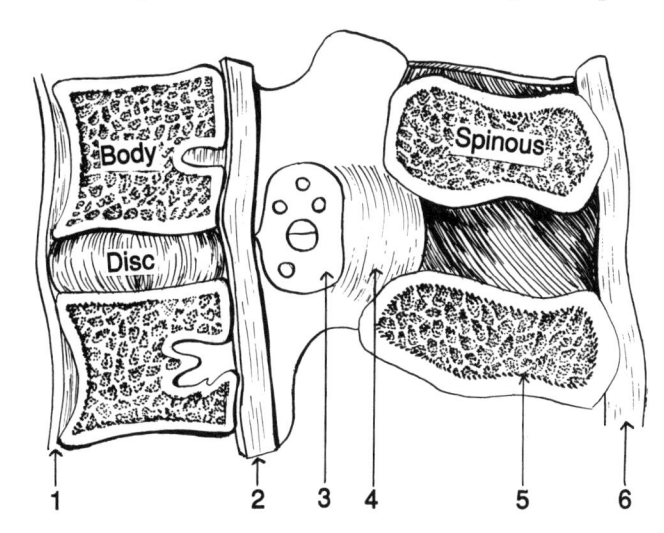

1. Ant. Long. Ligt.   2. Post. Long. Ligt.
3. Foramen/Contents   4. Ligamentum Flavum
5. Interspinous Ligt.   6. Supraspinous Ligt.

Figure 2–1

cess, with the interspinal and supraspinal ligament.

Tissues found within the intervertebral foramen are the spinal nerve root with its sheath, the recurrent meningeal nerve, blood vessels, both arteries and veins, lymphatics, and connective and fatty tissues.

This motor unit with its connecting parts is not a static entity, but moves in the ranges of the motions mentioned, and also moves in small increments day and night that are scarcely perceived by the individual.

In studying this manual it will become apparent that injury or reaction primarily affects two areas of this functional unit. The lower areas most often injured or reactive are the 5th lumbar segment and sacrum, which constitute the two parts of the lumbosacral joint. The second area is found in the thoracolumbar region, including the 11th and 12th thoracic segments and the 1st lumbar. These form the 11th and 12th thoracic motor unit, and the 12th thoracic/1st lumbar motor unit. The frequency of injury or reaction occurs twice as frequently at the thoracolumbar level as at the lumbosacral area.[2]

Joint injury or reaction can occur to tissues in or outside the motor unit. Neural tissues injured within the motor unit can cause structures found outside this unit to react, although they might not be involved in the injury per se. When the condition is uncontrolled, or in cases of permanent spinal lesions, permanent damage to these tissues can occur due to continued neural reaction. Injury to the tissues within the intervertebral foramen may affect the nerve tissues by direct or indirect neural trauma. This neural trauma or reaction is the cause of the tissue reaction outside of the intervertebral foramen. The injured level may affect adjacent levels because the nerve root, spinal nerve, and peripheral nerve are parts of the same nerve fiber. Injury to these nerve fibers may result from injury to the connective tissue or vascular supply at the nerve fiber. Changes in the blood flow may reduce available oxygen to the cell and can cause edema due to changes in cell permeability. Chemical changes are found to occur in some cases, causing a tissue electrolyte imbalance, leading to pain.[3] Changes other than nerve irritation develop, due to the biochemical imbalance resulting from reduced motion caused by the subluxation. The matrix changes, due to altered biochemical action, resulting in scar tissue that adheres to the articular surfaces.[4] All these changes occurring to the region of the foramen are injuries less than a dislocation lesion, and include injury to the vascular, neural, and other soft tissue at that area.

Tissues outside the foramen that are injured or reactive with potential injury are the supporting tissues and tissues that produce motion (see Figs. 2–2, 2–3, 2–4, and 2–5).

The deep muscles of the back such as the semispinalis, multifidus, rotatores, interspinales, and intertransversarii, which act to extend, laterally flex, and rotate the spine, can and do become involved when spinal lesions become reactive. All muscles that are part of the sacrospinalis muscle (Fig. 2–2), which connects to the pelvis, vertebrae,

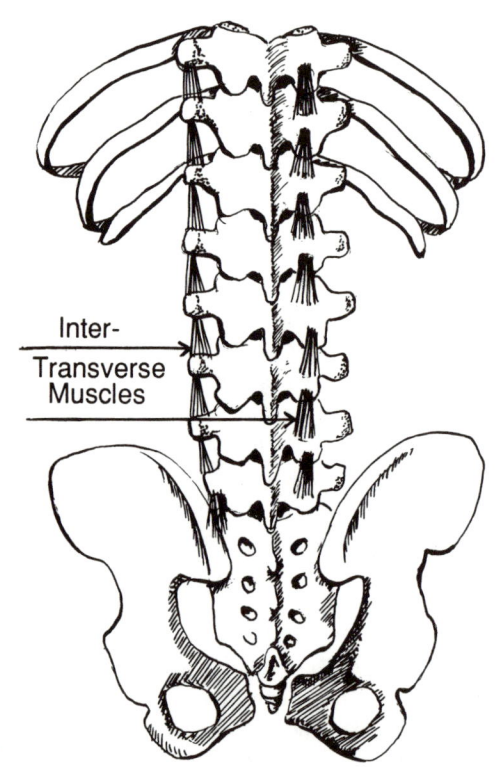

Figure 2–2

sacrum, and ribs, play their part in low back/leg pain syndromes by contraction, should that control be needed to act as a protective mechanism in the form of spinal splinting, when a lesion is present.[5]

If we investigate some of the deeper muscles of the back, we find that they differ in length and attachments and appear capable of antalgic contraction to a varying degree, depending upon the need.

The sacrospinalis is attached to the sacrum at one end and to the 11th and 12th thoracic vertebrae at the other. Some fibers from its broad base extend upward to attach to several of the lower ribs (see Fig. 2–3). The longissimus thoracis attaches to the transverse and accessory processes of the lumbar vertebrae (see No. 1 Fig. 2–4).

The multifidus has different length fibers that extend between 2nd, 3rd, 4th, and 5th vertebrae, which extend and rotate the spine. This muscle is aided by the rotatores, with fibers from the trans-

ANATOMY OF THE SPINE   11

verse process of one vertebra attaching to the spinous process of the adjacent vertebra. The intertransversarii supply fibers between the transverse processes at the thoracolumbar junction that bend the spine in a lateral position. (The attachments of all low back muscles and ligaments, both at the bottom and the top, can be seen in vivid color in the *Manual of Medicine* by Jiri Dvorak and Vaclav Dvorak.)[6]

The quadratus lumborum is an important muscle in lateral body flexion and comes into play following spinal injury in some low back cases, holding the body to one side in a protective manner. Its lower attachment at the iliac crest frequently becomes painful even when the muscle is mildly active (see Fig. 2–5: 1. deep layer; 2. superficial layers).[7]

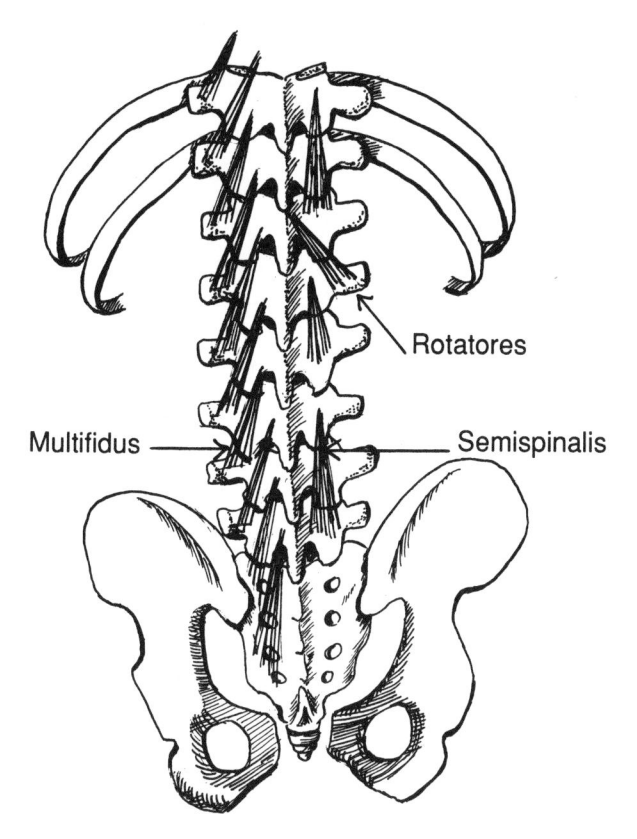

Figure 2–3

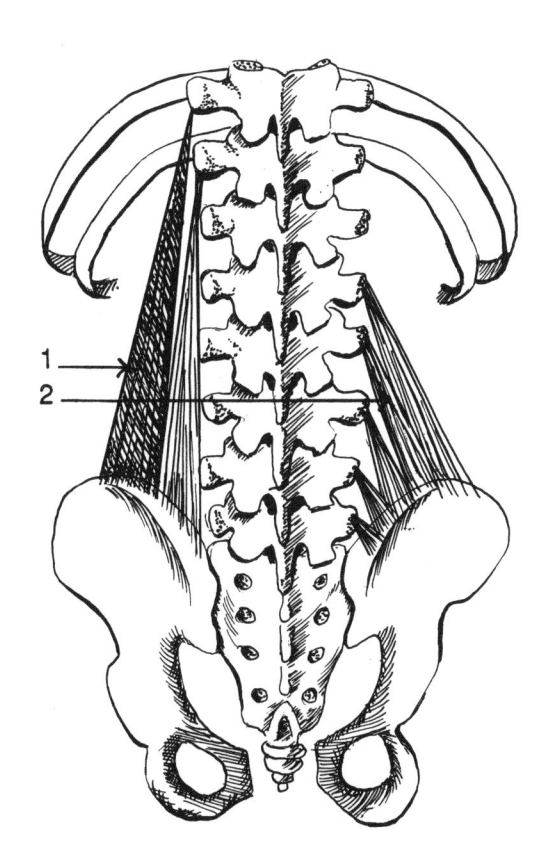

Figure 2–4

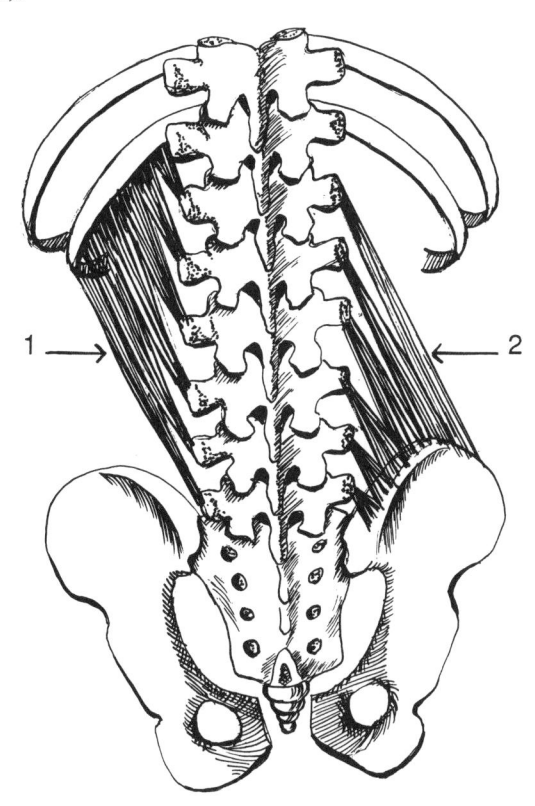

Figure 2–5

The interspinal and supraspinal ligaments are highly susceptible to injury and reaction, particularly at the level of the lumbosacral joint.[8] The supraspinal ligament seems to be the primary ligament injured or reactive. Its superficial fibers extend over the 3rd or 4th vertebrae, whereas the deeper fibers connect to the 2nd or 3rd vertebral segments. The deepest fibers merge with the interspinal ligaments and attach to two segments. This ligament also merges with other fascia at the lumbar area. The ligamental area most often involved in causing a major pain syndrome appears to be found at the lumbosacral joint.

In discussion of the nervous system related to low back/leg pain, it is important to be constantly aware that two primary nerve divisions of this system are present, and that either or both can be affected by injury, reaction to injury, and joint pathology.[9]

These two divisions are the posterior primary neural rami and anterior primary neural rami. Both divisions contribute to low back/leg pain, but the reasons may often be different.

Posterior Primary Rami

The meningeal nerve is a small, recurring branch from the posterior nerve root. It reenters the vertebral canal to supply nerve fibers to the vertebrae, ligaments, and blood vessels (see Fig. 2–6). These blood vessels supply nutrients, oxygen, and so on, and waste products are removed by this system. There is no hard evidence that this nerve is responsible for tissue reaction away from the spinal segments. The possibility that neural reaction from this nerve when injured may cause further response and irritation to other members of the posterior primary rami must be considered, however.

Continued irritation to the posterior primary rami by injury or disease may cause a reaction to muscles and ligaments outside the spinal motor units, most often as a protective mechanism (see Fig. 2–6).

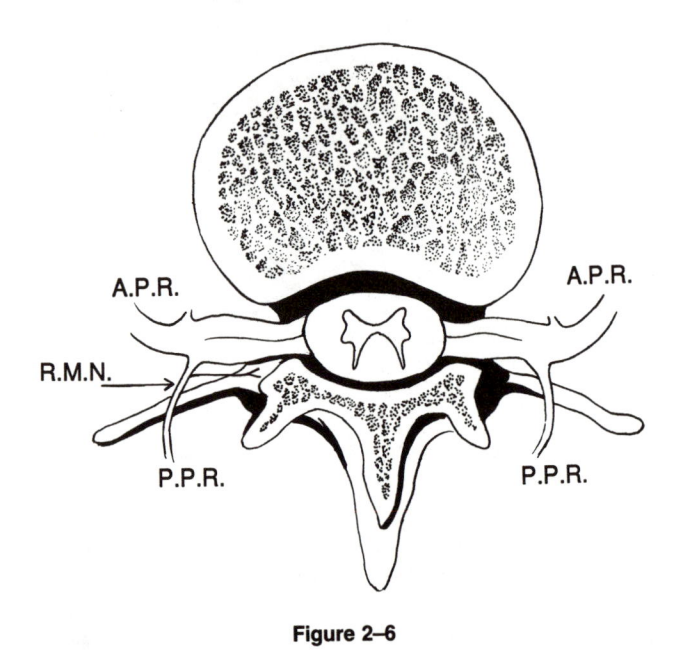

thus causing the pain syndromes that arise from it. (Refer to the chapter on the pain mechanism.)

Branches of the posterior rami turn backward to supply the skin and muscles of the back. The thoracic medial cutaneous branches extend downward as low as the iliac crest. The lumbar medial branches run close to the spine and end in the multifidus muscle. Lateral branches extend as low as the buttock and supply the sacrospinalis muscle. The sacral nerves are small, and supply the lower end of the multifidus muscle and the skin over the posterior portion of the buttock.

Anterior Primary Rami

The anterior primary rami is composed of two major neural groups creating pain syndromes at areas remote from the spine. It is essential that these two groups be separated for the recognition of the pain syndromes associated with each group, but also of the spinal level involved in the injury or reaction and the plexus involved causing those pain syndromes.

The two neural groups are the lumbar and sacral plexuses; each plexus contains certain nerves that, when injured or reactive, cause pain syndromes. Understanding the anatomy and pathology of these two neural groups opens the door to a better understanding of associated pain syndromes found in low back, pelvis, and leg pain cases.[2]

Lumbar Plexus Nerves
(Note only those listed in Fig. 2–7.)

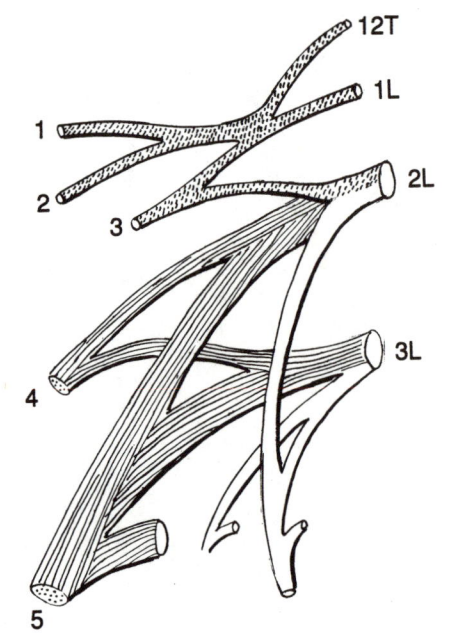

Figure 2–6

Irritation and response from the posterior primary rami can extend to the anterior primary rami,

Figure 2–7

- 12th Thoracic nerve (12T)
- 1st Lumbar nerve (1L)
- Iliohypogastric nerve (1)
- Ilioinguinal nerve (2)
- Genitofemoral nerve (3)
- Lateral femoral nerve (4)
- Femoral nerve (5)
- (Saphenous and/or lower-sural nerves connection)

The 4th lumbar spinal nerve plays an important role in either or both the lumbar and sacral plexuses. Its principal local reaction appears, however, to be associated with the sacral plexus. It is shown separated because of its dual relationship (see Fig. 2–8).

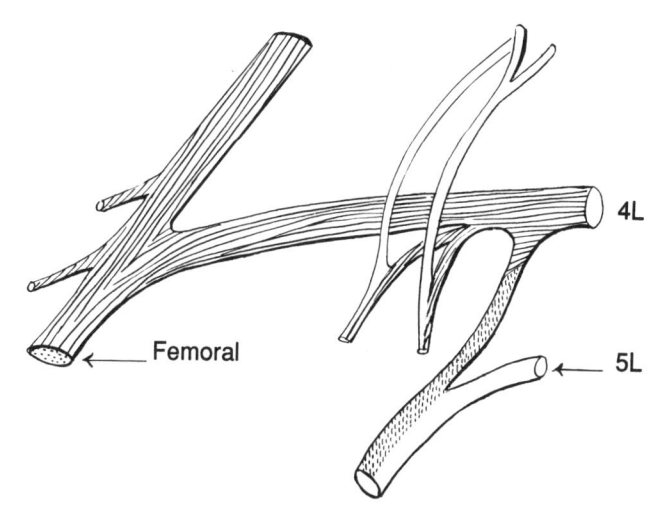

Figure 2–8

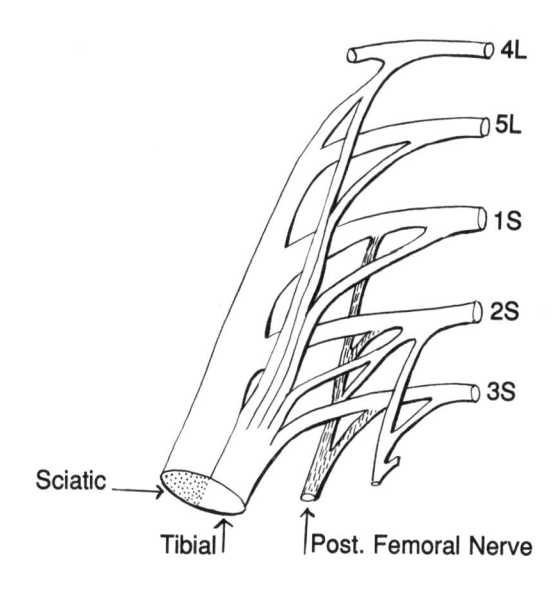

Figure 2–9

Sacral Plexus Nerves

- Great sciatic nerve
- Posterior femoral nerve
  (Saphenous or sural nerves)

Because most pain syndromes are reflected by cutaneous neural distribution, and not by dermatome areas, it is wise for the chiropractor to study various anatomy texts and become familiar with the cutaneous neural pain zones (see Fig. 2–9).

REFERENCES

1. Gray H: Gray's Anatomy 30th ed. Philadelphia, Lea & Febiger, 1984;p.347
2. Thomas JE: Classification of low back/leg pain syndromes, Part 3. *FCA Journal* January–February:39, 1986
3. Dishman R: Review of the literature supporting a scientific basis for the chiropractic subluxation complex. *JMPT* 8(3):163, 1985
4. Dishman R: Review of the literature supporting a scientific basis for the chiropractic subluxation complex. *JMPT* 8(3):163, 1985
5. Wood L: Acute locked facet syndrome and its treatment by manipulation under local periarticular anesthesia—Part 1: Clinical perspective and pilot study proposal. *JMPT* 7(4):211, 1984
6. Dvorak J, Dvorak V: General overview and list of the different muscles. In *Manual Medicine* Stuttgart-New York, Thieme-Stratton Inc., 1984;pp.49–126
7. Gray H: *Gray's Anatomy,* 30th ed. Philadelphia, Lea & Febiger, 1984;p.498
8. Thomas JE: Classification of low back/leg pain syndromes, Part 5. *FCA Journal* July–August:32, 1986
9. Rydevik B, Brown M, Lundburg G: Pathoanatomy and Pathophysiology of nerve root compression. *Spine* 9(1):7, 1984
10. Thomas JE: Classification of low back/leg pain syndromes, Part 3. *FCA Journal.* January–February:37, 1986

Chapter 3

Nerves to the Low Back, Pelvis, and Legs

DERMATOME VERSUS CUTANEOUS PAIN AREAS

In considering the nervous system and its relationship to pain syndromes, certain concepts that have existed for many years must be evaluated. Efforts have repeatedly been made to classify low back/leg pain as dermatome in origin, following dermatome patterns. Distortion of the pain area as described by the patient has resulted in order that this concept be followed. The greatest fault appears to be caused by inaccurate procedures for the determination of pain areas, which are now hopefully corrected.

Using the dermatome patterns, the spinal nerve level thought to be involved by injury or nerve reaction is different from the spinal levels found when the true pain areas are determined. Pain areas from the anterior primary rami closely follow the cutaneous nerve distribution as shown in almost all anatomy texts. Pain syndromes found in the low back region are also within the boundaries of the cutaneous nerves and reflect pain to underlying tissues at that area. Disc lesions do occur, severe damage and injury can result to nerve roots involving dermatomes; this condition is, however, only found in a small percentage of low back/leg pain cases.

NERVE AND NERVE GROUPS AND THEIR SPINAL LEVEL

The low back is a complex, multisegmental, universal joint capable of flexion, extension, lateral bending, and rotation. It differs from other universal joints because its motivating power source lies within the joint. This power impulse is transmitted via nerves that exist between each segment of the joint, stimulating muscle for this motion.

In considering the nerve supply for low back/leg pain, it is important to be aware that there are eight major pain syndromes. The purpose in the examination of the nervous system is to determine which nerves or nerve groups connect the spinal level of the power source to the pain syndromes and, if possible, to determine how this connection functions.

The primary symptom, pain, is in itself a warning and also a protective mechanism.[1,2] Tissues react in either case. Low back muscles begin to ache if the body remains in a cramped position too long. In severe cases, muscle splinting will be the body's reaction to prevent further damage.

The question is, which tissue of the low back is involved that can cause or invoke pain, has a constant pattern, can affect one or more areas, and can influence separate pain areas? The answer must be that no known single tissue found in the low back is adequately complex or selective to be responsible. For the present, the only common denominator for pain syndromes is that each syndrome is supplied by separate nerves, or nerve groups.

The principal nerve or nerve groups that supply each pain syndrome are as follows: (note drawing in Fig. 3–1).

- *Paraspinal:* dorsal primary rami of the spinal nerves[3]
- *Lumbar:* dorsal primary rami of the spinal nerves. Dorsal division of the 12th thoracic spinal nerve[4]
- *Gluteal:* dorsal primary rami of the 1st—2nd—3rd lumbar nerves;[5] (superior cluneal nerves)[6]
- *Thomas:* triangle portion—lateral cutaneous branch of the 12th thoracic nerve;[7] second portion—lateral cutaneous branch of the iliohypogastric nerve
- *Inguinal:* Upper portion—12th thoracic nerve—iliohypogastric nerves;[8] lower portion—iliohypogastric and ilioinguinal nerve
- *Anterior femoral:* anterior cutaneous branches of

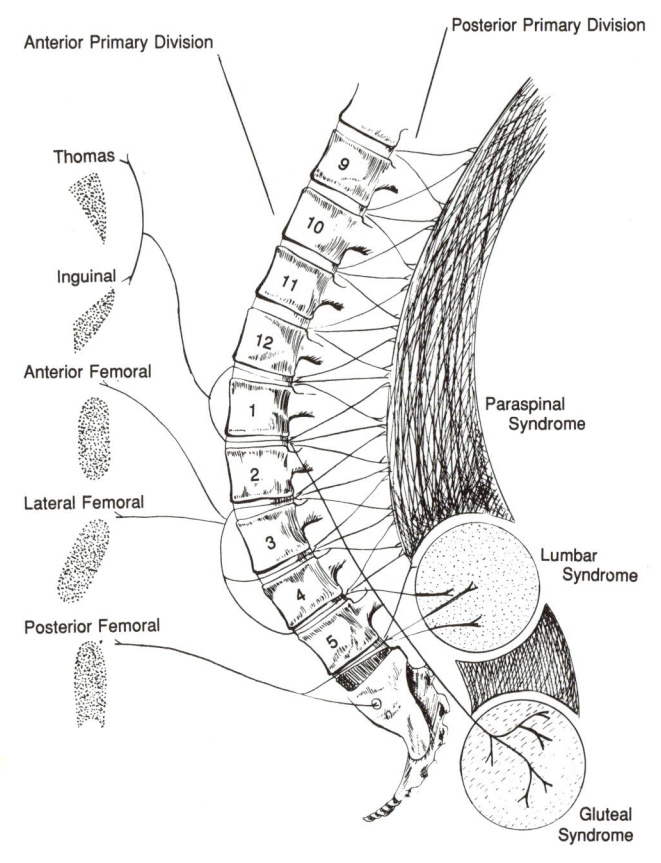

Figure 3–1

the femoral nerve;[9] (intermediate and medial cutaneous)[10]
- *Lateral femoral:* lateral femoral cutaneous nerve[11]
- *Posterior femoral:* posterior femoral cutaneous nerve.[12–13]

The nerve supplies described are the primary and obvious neural linkages to pain syndromes. There is, however, a less conspicuous neurologic connection that will become apparent as discussion progresses.

Reactive Tissue Resulting from Neural Response

To evaluate pain syndromes and their nerve supplies it is necessary to consider which tissue is injured, and the nature of that tissue's mode of reaction. It was previously mentioned that the spinal nerve root is vulnerable to injury at its exit from the spine. Thus, it can be anticipated that protective reaction will occur at the level of injury by those tissues best able to provide this protection, which can respond concurrently with the injury. The tissue that can best protect each nerve root is the muscle group responsible for spinal motion at that level, which may extend beyond that level if required.

Particularly from the 12th thoracic to the sacrum, the spine is well-endowed with muscles of varied lengths, capable of causing segmental immobilization.[14] Even directional immobilization is possible for the tranversospinal groups.[15] If an injury or tissue reaction involves more than one vertebral level, there will be sufficient muscle groups for the necessary protective response. The primary nerve supply for these muscles are the posterior primary rami, which are found at each nerve root level (see Fig. 3–2).[16]

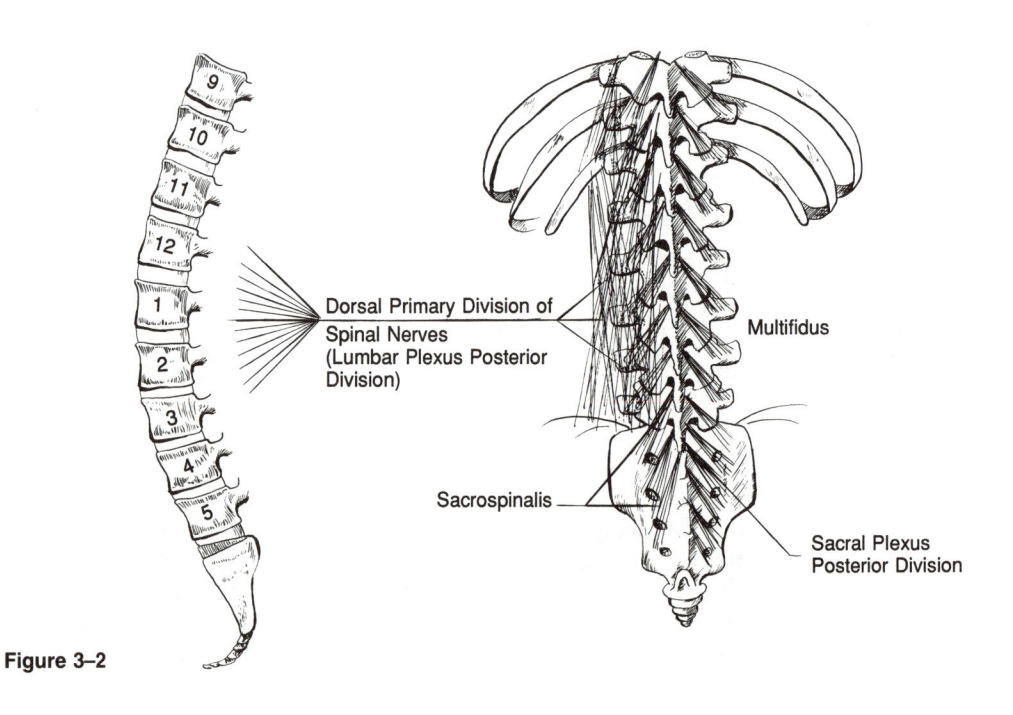

Figure 3–2

NERVES TO THE LOW BACK, PELVIS, AND LEGS   17

These nerves function as a group in spinal motion and they are capable of working in unison for the protection of multiple nerve root injury or potential injury.

IMPORTANT: The muscle contraction does not indicate injury to the muscle. The contraction is antalgic splinting and evidence of this splinting may be found by the spinal segmental examination. In severe cases, the contraction is great enough that the body may be pulled to one side. If this occurs, both the posterior and anterior primary rami are activated (see Fig. 3–3).[17]

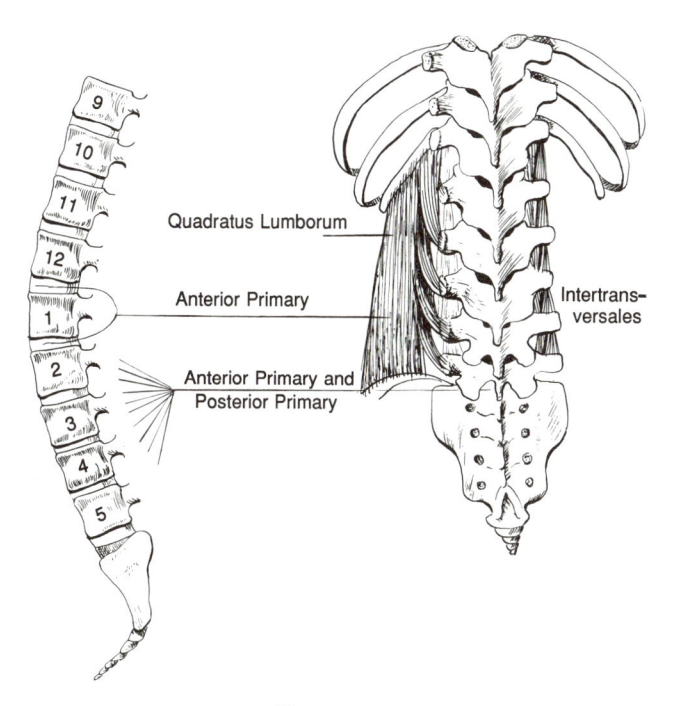

Figure 3–3

The distribution and severity of pain will depend upon the muscular response required for protection. This reaction constitutes an acute protective state and will continue until healing or a body compromise takes place. If the injury is resolved by treatment or natural repair, the affair is ended. When the normal state is not achieved, tissue will change into a pathologic state in an attempt to stabilize the joint for permanent protection.[18] When this change is completed, the muscles reduce their acute state to a chronic low-grade permanent status. Future injuries would reactivate this cycle. During the quiescent period, the patient may be relatively pain free. The previous information refers to the basic reason for pain found in the low back region. This includes the paraspinal and lumbar pain syndromes.

Posterior Primary Rami

The posterior primary rami (dorsal primary nerve division) from the thoracic and lumbar divisions supply muscles and the skin of the back and extend downward to the buttocks. Via the medial and lateral branches, this division supplies muscles such as the semispinalis, multifidus, transversospinales, longissimus, iliocostalis, and sacrospinalis. The dorsal division of the sacral nerves are smaller, and they end at the multifidus muscle. Various small branches supply the skin over the sacrum and coccyx and extend to the medial portion of the buttocks.

The gluteal syndrome appears to be caused by irritation to branches from the superior cluneal nerves. These nerves arise from the posterior primary rami. The root levels for these nerves are the 1st, 2nd, and 3rd lumbar, respectively (see Fig. 3–4).

Occasionally, there is some underlying tenderness to the gluteal muscles. Aided by upper sacral nerves, nerve fibers from the 4th and 5th lumbar spinal levels innervate the gluteal group. The presence or absence of gluteal muscle pain does not change the pain pattern, nor does the pain appear consistent when the 4th or 5th lumbar nerve is injured (see Fig. 3–4). Fibers from the 4th lumbar, and possibly from the 5th may, in rare cases, reinforce the cluneal nerves.[19–20]

The paraspinal, lumbar, and gluteal pain syndromes are caused by injury or reaction from the posterior primary rami.

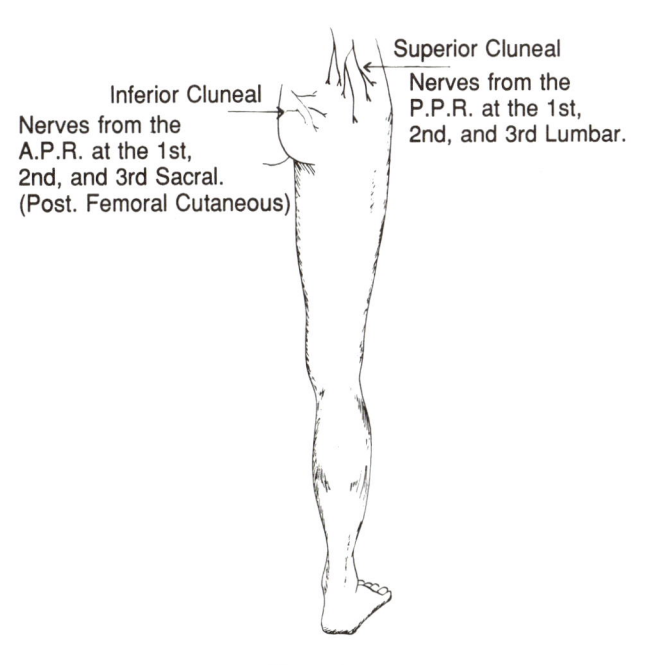

Figure 3–4

Anterior Primary Rami

The anterior primary rami (ventral primary nerve division) primarily supply muscles and skin away from the spine.

Changes in normal neural anatomy may effect some differences related to the location of pain areas from spinal injuries or reaction. The following information mentions a few of these anatomical variations.

The lumbar plexus arises from the 1st, 2nd, 3rd, and a large portion of the 4th lumbar nerves.[21] The smaller portion of the 4th lumbar nerve joins with the 5th lumbar nerve to form the lumbosacral trunk. There are variations to this major nerve supply in the following manner. When the 3rd lumbar nerve is the lowest to supply fibers to the lumbosacral trunk, it is called the *high* or *prefixed plexus*. When the 5th lumbar is the lowest nerve to supply nerve fibers to the lumbosacral trunk, it is called the *low* or *postfixed plexus*. We find that the 12th thoracic and 1st lumbar nerves contribute to form the ilioinguinal nerve. The genitofemoral nerve is formed by portions of the 1st and 2nd lumbar roots. Several textbooks indicate that communication between the 12th thoracic and iliohypogastric may not always be present.[22] They also state that considerable variation in neuroanatomy may be found at the iliohypogastric, ilioinguinal, genitofemoral, and the femoral branches.

Pain syndromes caused by injury or reaction to the anterior primary rami are the inguinal, Thomas, anterior femoral, lateral femoral, and the posterior femoral syndrome.

The possibility appears that anatomical differences play a part in the existence of the Thomas and inguinal syndromes (see Figs. 3–5, 3–6).

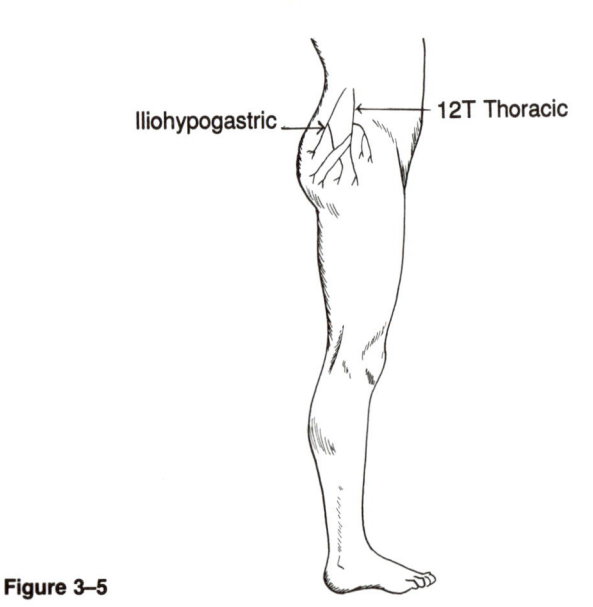

Figure 3–5

Figure 3–6

The 12th thoracic, iliohypogastric, and ilioinguinal appear, as a group, to be responsible for the inguinal and Thomas pain syndromes.

Most frequently, the first lumbar nerve receives a branch from the 12th thoracic, and when present, it forms the iliohypogastric nerve. This nerve divides into two branches, the anterior and lateral cutaneous nerves. The lateral cutaneous branches of both the 12th thoracic and iliohypogastric appear to be responsible for the posterior pain area of the Thomas syndrome, in an inverse proportion. They supply the skin at the gluteal region posterior to that area supplied by the 12th thoracic nerve, which is the smaller portion of the Thomas pain syndrome. The anterior branch of the iliohypogastric nerve supplies the upper portion of the inguinal pain syndrome at the hypogastric area.

The ilioinguinal nerve communicates with the iliohypogastric. These nerves appear to be responsible for the lower portion of the inguinal pain syndrome. There is probably an association with the genitofemoral in this pain syndrome, particularly that portion arising from the first lumbar nerve.[23] A minor pain syndrome that arises from the genitofemoral nerve when injury or reaction occurs to that nerve is known to exist.

In the leg region, there are three pain syndromes whose nerve supplies also arise from the ventral primary rami. The anterior femoral syndrome is supplied by the anterior cutaneous branches of the femoral nerve (see Fig. 3–7).[24]

These branches are the intermediate and medial cutaneous nerves. The intermediate nerve divides into two branches and supplies the anterior portion of the thigh. At the top of the thigh, it communicates with the genitofemoral nerve, and at the knee with branches of the saphenous nerve. The communication at the knee between the genitofemoral nerve and branches from the saphenous nerve forms another minor pain syndrome that is occasionally present without any other pain to the limb; it is difficult to differentiate it from knee problems. When no pathology or injury is evident related to the knee and all examination procedures exclude

NERVES TO THE LOW BACK, PELVIS, AND LEGS   19

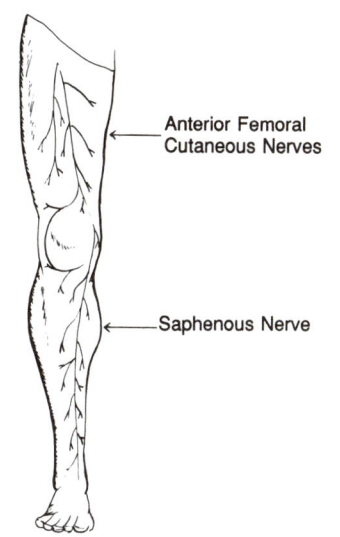

Figure 3–7

the knee joint, this minor pain syndrome should be considered, particularly when the spinal segmental examination indicates a reactive rating at the thoracolumbar segments. The medial cutaneous nerve is not involved often enough that this pain syndrome be classified as a major one. It has to be considered a minor pain syndrome because the medial side of the thigh becomes painful only occasionally.

Both branches from the femoral nerve communicate with the saphenous nerve and, as a result, either or both may contribute to pain extending to the medial side of the leg. The pain from this nerve may extend from the knee downward, including the anterior or medial portion of the lower leg, to the ankle, and may even include the great toe. It is not common, but this area of pain, caused by a spinal lesion of the femoral nerve, may only involve this area, or small portions of it.

The nerve supply for the lateral femoral syndrome is the anterior and posterior branches of the lateral femoral cutaneous nerve (see Fig. 3–8).[25]

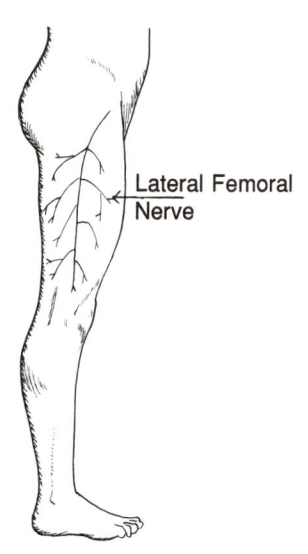

Figure 3–8

This nerve arises from the second and third lumbar nerves and is also found in the ventral primary nerve division. The anterior branch supplies the skin over the anterior and lateral portions of the thigh, but the posterior branch appears to be the branch causing the pain over the lateral area of the thigh from the trochanter to the middle of the thigh. This is the area of complaint described by the patient for this pain syndrome. Pain to the knee is occasionally found when this pain syndrome is present.

The posterior femoral nerve supplies the posterior portion of the thigh from the lower buttocks, continuing downward to, and including, the back of the knee, and communicates with the sural nerve via the sural branches of the posterior femoral nerve (see Fig. 3–9).

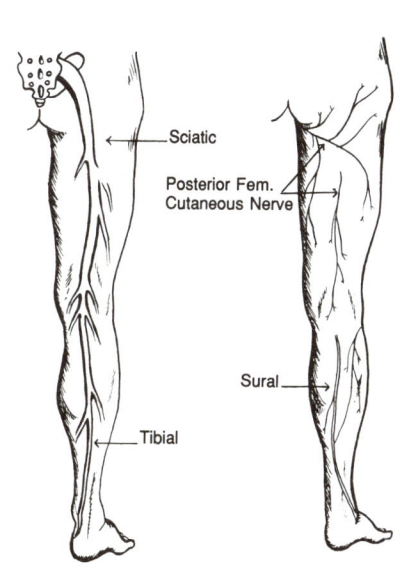

Figure 3–9

The sural nerve supplies the posterior lateral portion of the leg, portions of the heel, lateral ankle, and toes. Spinal roots supplying this nerve are the 1st, 2nd, and 3rd sacral.[26–27]

One synonym for the posterior femoral cutaneous nerve is the *small sciatic nerve*. It might be argued that, when injured, this nerve is still a sciatic case. It is unfortunate that the great and small sciatic nerves have not been separated relative to posterior leg pain. The fault lies in the absence of a differential diagnostic procedure and the interpretation of existing examination procedures. This information will be discussed in Chapter 15, referring to posterior femoral pain syndromes. Any tissues of the pelvis and leg region are supplied by fibers from the 5th lumbar nerve root. The gluteal maximus, obturator, and gemellus muscles are in close proximity to the posterior femoral nerve, and they receive fibers from the 5th lumbar root. It may be possible that these muscles, or their nerve fibers, or both, play a part in causes of posterior femoral pain.[28] It is also well-known that, when injured, nerve fibers can react at adjacent spinal levels.[29-31] This metamerism is probably the primary cause of posterior femoral pain.

Nerve Supply to Each Syndrome

We have now discussed the nerve supply for each syndrome. In reviewing the spinal level involved with each nerve or nerve group for the syndromes it is necessary to consider the following.

1. The paraspinal and lumbar pain syndromes are supplied by the dorsal primary at each spinal level from the 12th thoracic to the 5th lumbar.
2. The gluteal syndrome is supplied also by the dorsal primary rami of the 1st, 2nd, and 3rd lumbar, arising from the same spinal levels.
3. The Thomas and inguinal pain syndromes are caused from injury at the 12th thoracic and 1st lumbar root.
4. Supplying fibers to the lateral femoral syndrome, the lateral femoral cutaneous nerve arises from the 2nd and 3rd lumbar nerve.
5. Supplied by branches of the femoral nerve, the anterior femoral pain syndrome arises from the 2nd, 3rd, and 4th lumbar levels.
6. The posterior femoral syndrome, involving the posterior femoral nerves, appears to be supplied from the 5th lumbar level, via metamerism.

After reviewing the spinal levels and considering the overlapping nerve supply related to pain syndromes, it is not difficult to understand the problems associated with the differential diagnosis of low back/leg pain cases. This point has probably been reached by other physicians in low back/leg pain research and scrapped because of this apparent maze.

Knowledge of the pain syndromes, their precise locations, with the major nerve supply to each of these areas and coupled with the spinal segmental examination and its findings, now enables an effective differential diagnosis of low back/leg pain cases. The following chapters in this manual will show how these varying factors related to low back/leg pain can be connected and evaluated.

REFERENCES

1. Wood J: Acute locked facet syndrome and its treatment by manipulation under local periarticular anesthesia—Part 1: Clinical perspective and pilot study proposal. *JMPT* 7(4):211, 1984
2. Pressman RH, Nickles S: Neurophysiological and nutritional considerations of pain control. *JMPT* 7(4):219, 1984
3. Hamilton WJ (ed): *Textbook of Human Anatomy*, 2nd ed. St. Louis MO, CV Mosby Co, 1976;p.138
4. Gray H: *Gray's Anatomy*, 30th ed. Philadelphia, Lea & Febiger, 1984;p.1198
5. Hamilton WJ (ed): *Textbook of Human Anatomy*, 2nd ed. St. Louis MO, CV Mosby Co, 1976;p.638
6. Netter F: *Atlas of Human Anatomy*, 2nd ed. Summit NJ, CIBA Pharmaceuticals, 1989;Plate 513
7. Gray H: *Gray's Anatomy*, 30th ed. Philadelphia, Lea & Febiger, 1984;p.1223
8. Hamilton WJ (ed): *Textbook of Human Anatomy*, 2nd ed. St. Louis MO, CV Mosby Co, 1976;p.639
9. Gray H: *Gray's Anatomy*, 30th ed. Philadelphia, Lea & Febiger, 1984;p.1229
10. Netter F: *Atlas of Human Anatomy*, 2nd ed. Summit NJ, CIBA Pharmaceuticals, 1989;Plate 506
11. Gray H: *Gray's Anatomy*, 30th ed. Philadelphia, Lea & Febiger, 1984;p.1229
12. Gray H: *Gray's Anatomy*, 30th ed. Philadelphia, Lea & Febiger, 1984;p.1237
13. Netter F: *Atlas of Human Anatomy*, 2nd ed. Summit NJ, CIBA Pharmaceuticals, 1989;Plate 506
14. Good AB: Spinal joint blocking. *JMPT* 8(1):1, 1985
15. Dvorak J, Dvorak V: *Manual Medicine*. Stuttgart-New York, Thieme-Stratton Inc, 1984;p.65
16. Netter F: *Atlas of Human Anatomy*, 2nd ed. Summit NJ, CIBA Pharmaceuticals, 1989;Plate 156
17. Gray H: *Gray's Anatomy*, 30th ed. Philadelphia, Lea & Febiger, 1984;p.498
18. Good AB: Spinal joint blocking. *JMPT* 8(1):1, 1985
19. Gray H: *Gray's Anatomy*, 30th ed. Philadelphia, Lea & Febiger, 1984;p.1236
20. Netter F: *Atlas of Human Anatomy*, 2nd ed. Summit NJ, CIBA Pharmaceuticals, 1989;Plate 513
21. Gray H: *Gray's Anatomy*, 30th ed. Philadelphia, Lea & Febiger, 1984;p.1226
22. Gray H: *Gray's Anatomy*, 30th ed. Philadelphia, Lea & Febiger, 1984;p.1229
23. Gray H: *Gray's Anatomy*, 30th ed. Philadelphia, Lea & Febiger, 1984;p.1223
24. Gray H: *Gray's Anatomy*, 30th ed. Philadelphia, Lea & Febiger, 1984;p.1231
25. Gray H: *Gray's Anatomy*, 30th ed. Philadelphia, Lea & Febiger, 1984;p.1237
26. Netter F: *Atlas of Human Anatomy*, 2nd ed. Summit NJ, CIBA Pharmaceuticals, 1989;Plate 508
27. Gray H: *Gray's Anatomy*, 30th ed. Philadelphia, Lea & Febiger, 1984;p.1237
28. Gray H: *Gray's Anatomy*, 30th ed. Philadelphia, Lea & Febiger, 1984;p.1238
29. Best CH, Taylor NB: *The Physiological Basis of Medical Practice*, 4th ed. Baltimore, Williams & Wilkins, 1945;p.847
30. Turek SL: *Orthopedic Principles and Their Application*, 3rd ed. Philadelphia, JB Lippincott, 1959;p.223
31. Hoppenfeld S: *Orthopedic Neurology*. Philadelphia, JB Lippincott, 1977;p.67

Chapter 4

Spinal Lesions

SPINAL LESIONS CAUSING LOW BACK, PELVIC, AND LEG PAIN SYNDROMES

There is no scientific evidence that gross pathological changes are the primary cause of all low back/leg pain cases. There is, however, growing evidence that spinal lesions less severe than a luxation are not only the major cause of low back/leg pain, but are responsible for pain at other areas of the body. This chapter is about that lesion.

Many articles have been written about the spinal lesion. Some authors use the term subluxation; others describe this condition as joint dysfunction or abnormal joint motion. Dorland's dictionary describes a subluxation as an incomplete or partial dislocation. The term *dysfunction* refers to a partial disturbance, impairment, or abnormality of the functioning organ. The author prefers to use disrelation as a description. The term *relation* means the way in which one thing is related to another. Disrelation indicates that the normal relation between two objects is impaired. Dr. Good discusses joint bind, locking, fixation, and restriction.[1] As presently accepted, no single term appears to fit or include all the actions and reactions that occur to a spinal joint and other associated tissue. Many authors have described this lesion using different terminology, although it is obvious that they are discussing the same pathological entity.

Common to most articles and text that describe this entity is a fluent description regarding pathological changes to the spine and its joints. In dealing with spinal problems, it is, of course, essential to be aware of all systemic or constitutional diseases that relate to bone and joints. Nonetheless, when a patient with low back/leg pain is examined and the average physician finds constitutional or degenerative joint pathology, diagnosis and treatment are often directed at that condition. It would be wiser to look further and explore the possibility of acute subluxation/disrelations that might actually be the basic cause of pain or disability.

Both chiropractic and medical physicians must be aware that joint disrelation of the spine may be one cause of spinal and nerve pathology. The basic problem may be, however, how to separate subluxation/disrelation from other pathologies and how to diagnose it when no other pathology is evident.

Questions that need to be answered are:

- Does a subluxation/disrelation lesion exist, does it have a symptom complex and, if so, what are the symptoms?
- Can a spinal pathological condition cause a subluxation, and how might these conditions relate to one another?
- Can we prove that this subluxation/disrelation is changed, or that a beneficial result is caused by specific segmental manipulation?

Although included here the latter question is best answered in Chapter 19 of this manual. The treating physician who takes these questions into account is better equipped to identify the most effective treatment for each individual patient.

The existence of a subluxation was proven 34 years ago by L. A. Hadley.[2] He indicated that normal physiological movements cause an enlargement or encroachment of the spinal foramen, and that this finding must be considered when symptoms of nerve root pressure are present. He stated that mechanical pressure is too narrow a viewpoint, that strain and inflammation at the spinal exit could cause pressure symptoms. Degenerative nerve root changes were shown when these nerves were removed from their foramen at autopsy. This degeneration was caused by a subluxation lesion.

If we investigate the second edition of the A.M.A. *Guide to the Evaluation of Permanent Impairment*,[3] we find a small section designated for impairment factors in which a subluxation is diagnosed as reduced or unreduced. This small section is not comprehensive, as the purpose of this book is to provide those guidelines that can aid in evaluating an impairment rating, should it be indicated. In the final analysis it is, however, the responsibility of the doctor to examine each spinal segment and diagnose a subluxation, when present, and to rate its status. Every chiropractic physician is well aware of the Medicare codes and the list of associated pathologies that relate to a subluxation. The fact that a spinal subluxation/disrelation lesion can exist is not hypothetical.

In order that spinal joint lesions are understood, it is first necessary to know the nature of a lesion.

DEFINITION OF A LESION

A lesion is

Any pathological or traumatic discontinuity of tissue or loss of function of a part. (Dorland's Illustrated Medical Dictionary)

A joint lesion, when defined, includes any joint of the body, but the spinal joint is unique in that it not only functions as a joint related to motion, but is also designed as part of a unit that protects the spinal cord and associated nerve roots. Hence, the definition of the spinal joint is not only appropriate, but a requirement for this distinction.

Definition of a Subluxation/Disrelation Lesion

What is a subluxation? *It is an abnormal relationship, at the joint, between two bony structures, that is present during motion and the transitional stage, and that continues to exist in a static position. This disrelationship is a pathologic entity with tissue reaction as its sequel.*[4] *This pathologic entity can be disrelated both anatomically and physiologically, or both.*

The definition of a subluxation in this manual describes this generic lesion as simply as possible, and includes all basic information so that the elements of the definition can remain intact. Although physicians may know in their minds what this lesion is, a simple, concise, word structure should be available for everyone to understand.

1. The definition notes where the lesion exists: *At the joint between two bony structures.* This is uncomplicated and easily understood.
2. It also indicates its basic characteristics. This is answered in the following manner: "the disrelation is present during motion and the transitional stage, and continues to exist in a static position." Thus, the practitioner is able to visualize the range of motion from one point to another with the lesion existing during that period of motion; when the motion stops, the lesion being still present, remains present until some action changes its status.

The ramifications of this word usage become increasingly evident when it is considered associated with various forms of spinal treatment. Think of subluxation with this word usage and meaning during the following treatment procedures:

- Traction
- Massage
- Injections
- Pain killers
- Surgery
- Nonspecific manipulation

Unless the characteristics of the lesion are changed by some specific treatment to that joint, it will continue to exist, and this unfortunately is one major cause of chronic low back/leg pain.

3. This definition interprets the condition as a pathologic lesion that may sound superficially unnecessary; but benign lesions do exist and cause few or no symptoms.
4. As a pathological lesion, it must react adversely to the body. "This disrelationship is a pathological entity with tissue reaction as its sequel." In other words, it must cause certain tissues to react, thus creating a symptom complex.
5. The subluxation/disrelation pathological lesion has a sequel, if untended, or if beyond aid. The scientific references related to the sequel for this lesion are now found in abundance.
6. The definition of subluxation also indicates the immediate tissues involved in a generic sense. "This pathological entity can be disrelated both anatomically and/or physiologically." The subclassification refers to our present knowledge of these tissues.

Although flexible, our definition is sound and can be defended by the chiropractor and understood by those with average medical knowledge.

It is possible, of course, that a subluxation may exist in a form not presently understood or known. In order to provide provisions for this possible eventuality, the subluxation will be classified.

CLASSIFICATION OF THE SPINAL LESION

With their connecting parts, the two vertebrae act as a unit within the total. This unit is not a static entity. Flexion, extension, lateral bending, and rotation are the motions of the multiple motor units found in the spinal column. Each unit does contain, however, individual muscle groups and attachments that enable isolated antalgic muscle contraction for that unit, although the unit works within the whole. Each unit contributes to these motions in varying degrees, depending upon its location in the spinal column.

Any constitutional disease, birth defect, or injury that disturbs the smooth rhythmic motion of these units creates a subluxation. A pathological condition that changes the anatomical structure of bone or soft tissue associated with this unit also changes the functioning relationship of the unit.

An injury such as a vertebral body fracture can change the functioning relationship of the motor unit and cause a permanent subluxation. Because these subluxations exist within a pathological condition, they are classified as "secondary subluxations."

Secondary versus Primary Spinal Lesion

Many secondary subluxations may be dormant, pain free, or so minimal that they cause few problems if the patient uses some caution. As constitutional disease progresses, vertebral disrelation can occur slowly, allowing the body ample time to adjust to the abnormal condition. For example, a patient may live 50 years with a scoliosis containing several unit disrelationships before a reaction occurs, and then only following an injury. Even a previously unreduced subluxation that has become dormant may remain so until the right motion in sufficient force or the right angle of force causes it to react.

An injury with a delayed reaction would probably be a secondary subluxation. Previously injured tissue that has slowly changed its structure to comply with the injury enables it to become dormant or nonreactive and it no longer has the capability of reacting as normal healthy tissue. Even when the reaction is evident, the response may be far greater or less than would occur in normal tissue. This does not mean an immediate reaction is impossible; each case must be evaluated on its own.

The difference between a primary and secondary subluxation will be of importance because it has a bearing on the mode of treatment.

The reaction of a primary or first-time subluxation is sudden and intense. There are no inhibitions to healthy tissue and a protective response is immediate. A sudden unexpected force will cause a disrelationship, producing an immediate tissue reaction. Several delayed quick forces whether unexpected or deliberate, in the same direction, may cause a subluxation with immediate tissue reaction following the final insult. A steady maximum force may cause a segmental disrelation, particularly to the weakest joint or motor unit, followed by tissue reaction. A prolonged weaker force in the same direction may cause a milder form of subluxation, less than maximum, followed by a delayed or weaker reaction. Any combination of the above such as sudden changes in the direction of the force can produce the same results.[5]

The injured or deformed tissue in a secondary subluxation appears to react in a different fashion. The patient with an old, unreduced subluxation that has been dormant is susceptible to recurrences. These recurrences may appear in any form, from mild to severe and, seemingly, not always related to the precipitant force.

The secondary subluxation associated with a constitutional disease or deformity can also react at any time when additional stress, fatigue, strain, or further injury occurs. Considerable variation in the intensity of the reaction is possible. We must remember that the disrelationship may have existed in many cases for some period of time, its tissues having adjusted to the abnormal state. Subsequent changes will cause a reaction, depending upon the amount of further tissue injury and its ability to respond.

We now know that two types of subluxations occur. In order to better understand the subluxation lesion, let us classify it thus.[6]

1. A primary subluxation is a lesion caused by an injury or neural reaction to normal healthy tissue.
2. A secondary subluxation is a lesion that is a consequence of, or sequel to, previous pathology or injury. It is also subject to injury or neural reaction.

Both of these lesions may be found in an acute or chronic state. An acute lesion may become chronic and dormant, and in the future if injured again may have an acute reaction, although the lesion at that time would be classified as secondary. Joint changes due to constitutional disease, and so on, are a secondary subluxation lesion and they may be dormant or reactive. If dormant, they are also subject to further injury and neural reaction. Either or both these reactions can occur or be present at any motor unit of the spinal column.

To better understand the spinal subluxation, the subclassification including the known tissues involved are listed below.

Subclassification of a Subluxation/Disrelation Lesion

1. Trophic lesions
2. Vascular lesions
3. Neural lesions
4. Facet lesions
5. Disc lesions
6. Other soft tissues' lesions
7. Bone lesions (injury, disease, congenital, acquired)
8. Hypomobility of vertebral segments
9. Hypermobility of vertebral segments
10. Any combination of the above

Returning to the question of whether a subluxation causes a symptom and, if so, which symptom?—when the term "subluxation" is used, it is often not understood due to the lack of proper coding. Thus it is advantageous to change the question and ask whether an interspinal joint disrelationship causes symptoms, and if so, which symptoms? The question phrased in this manner may give a more accurate description of the injury. In any event, a subluxation, joint disrelation, or joint dysfunction is one and the same.

SYMPTOMS OF A SPINAL LESION

In the context of this book a symptom is defined as

> *A sign of the existence of a condition, especially a perceptible change from what is normal in the body or its functioning, indicating disease or injury.* (Oxford American Dictionary, 1980) (Dorland's Illustrated Medical Dictionary states about the same thing.)

If a pathological disrelationship is caused by injury to an extremity joint such as the knee or elbow, pain and limitation of motion are produced by injury or pathology.[7] Although no spinal nerve root is present at the elbow or knee, this does not negate a protective or tissue injury reaction. The spinal joint is no different; it also can react to tissue injury, and in a defensive manner.[8] The anterior spinal rami is not involved in the greatest percentage of spinal subluxations or spinal joint disrelations. Most muscles that react defensively are neurologically supplied by the posterior spinal rami. This neuromuscular system is responsible for spinal motion. Antalgic contraction is a protective muscular mechanism and is part of this system.

Although paraspinal antalgic contraction is part of the subluxation symptom complex, it may also be transitional.

During an acute primary or reactive secondary subluxation, antalgic contraction will be present. In old primary or secondary subluxation, it is likely that the reactive antalgic contractions are absent, and tissues will be fibrosed.[9] Variations of this symptom complex can occur from the onset of a primary subluxation to the old nonreactive subluxation. The average patient seeking chiropractic service is prompted by pain. This is particularly true for low back/leg pain. Hence, pain is part of a subluxation symptom complex. Pain, however, similar to antalgic contraction, does not always respond in a simple, uncomplicated manner. Injuries are variable; as a result, subluxations or joint disrelations range from mild to severe. The reactions should of course vary, depending upon the degree of insult. Because the reactions are pain and antalgic contraction, they too can range from mild to severe.

The degree of joint disrelation cannot, however, be rated by the tissue response in the form of pain or antalgic contraction. Even the amount of reaction may differ from one patient to another.

For the moment, setting aside any involvement of the anterior primary rami, it is appropriate to consider pain associated with joint disrelation due to immediate injury.

Response from the Posterior Primary Rami

A spinal joint is traumatized: disrelation occurs. The immediate effect is pain and muscle splinting, which is produced by muscles of the low back region, and is located at the level of the injured motor unit. A minimum of two vertebrae are involved in this splinting. When the 5th lumbar motor unit is injured, the sacrum becomes part of the splinted area.

So that no error or misconception occurs in reference to the low back, the 12th thoracic vertebra to the 5th lumbar is included; In many cases, the 10th and 11th thoracic must be considered within this group.[3] Any motor unit in this group may be injured, will respond by pain and paraspinal splinting to the spinal column at that level, and may range up or down from that level depending upon the severity of the injury. A disc or anterior primary nerve injury is not a requisite for the described reaction. The pain associated with this reaction may register as mild to highly reactive. Once antalgic contraction fixes the motor unit, the pain may become negligible unless the patient bends into the position that can further traumatize it, or cause reaction at the lesion. Pain, restricted motion, or both, is then apt to be experienced.

There are two areas of the low back that appear most susceptible to injury, namely the level of the 12th thoracic and, secondarily, the 5th lumbar motor unit. After examining 6000 spinal segments, spinal segmental examination procedures have shown that the 12th thoracic motor unit injury leads the 5th lumbar injuries 2:1. The statistical recording of 572 injured and reactive spinal motor units has found that they appear as shown in the following chart.

Vertebral motor unit	Number reactive
12th thoracic	427
4th lumbar	48
5th lumbar	185
other units	40

It should be obvious that some cases have more than one level involved. (Note: The importance of this will be discussed in Chapters 5 and 16). We now have two symptoms caused by a subluxation or joint disrelation:

1. Spinal protective antalgic contraction
2. Paraspinal pain resulting from joint injury and associated muscle contraction[10]

Response from the Anterior Primary Rami

To consider the anterior primary nerve rami, it is necessary to be aware of which pain area is being discussed, its frequency of occurrence, and identification of the nerve involved.

Only 27% of all low back/leg pain found in single pain syndromes results from injury to the anterior primary rami. The analysis and percentages are as follows:

Thomas syndrome	4%
Inguinal syndrome	4%
Anterior femoral syndrome	7%
Lateral femoral syndrome	7%
Posterior femoral syndrome	6%

The anterior primary rami at the 12th thoracic and 1st lumbar levels combine in many cases to form a neural linkage, the 12th thoracic–iliohyogastric–ilioinguinal and 1st lumbar. This nerve group acts as a unit in spinal motion. The two areas of pain, the Thomas and inguinal pain syndromes, appear to be a result of root injury or reaction to this neural linkage.[11] Because the 12th thoracic motor unit is involved in by far the greatest percentage of lumbar plexus injuries, the two vertebrae, the 12th thoracic and 1st lumbar, should be suspected as disrelated. No case in which the Thomas and inguinal syndromes are present, indicating a primary disc lesion, has come to this author's attention. If these pain syndromes are combined on a percentage basis, the resultant figure is 8% of all single-syndrome low back/leg pain patients.

The femoral and anterior femoral nerves arise from the lumbar plexus. The spinal segmental or motor unit levels for these nerves are the 2nd and 3rd lumbar vertebral levels and they appear responsible for the anterior and lateral femoral syndromes. Again, no evidence of a primary disc lesion has been found.

The 3rd lumbar motor unit appears to be the least affected by injury. The two reactive areas are the thoracolumbar region and the lumbosacral region. During the examination, the physician rarely finds muscle contraction breaking through the neutral 3rd lumbar unit. This leads to the belief that both femoral syndromes most often arise from irritation or inflammation of the 2nd lumbar nerve root.

The number of injuries to the 5th lumbar motor unit is secondary to the number of injuries occurring at the thoracolumbar junction. Of all low back pain, 28% is caused by a subluxation of the 5th lumbar motor unit, and in these cases only the posterior primary rami are involved. The anterior rami are injured in only 6% of all low back/leg pain cases at the 5th lumbar. This latter percentage appears to involve only the posterior femoral nerve, not the great sciatic nerve. The posterior femoral nerve arises from sacral levels 1, 2, and 3.

It is known that nerve roots carry fibers from adjacent nerve roots. Injury to the 5th lumbar anterior primary nerve carrying 1st sacral elements seems to be responsible for the posterior femoral syndrome.[12] It is well-known that nerve roots can be injured without pressure from a disc lesion. The mode of reaction is still not completely understood, but appears to be caused by changes to the vascular supply and tissue reaction in the form of inflammation with pathological tissue changes.[13] The subluxation or disrelation associated with a disc lesion is classified under the secondary subluxation. The disc lesion as a cause or effect of a subluxation must be labeled under pathological entities. A true disc herniation causes pressure symptoms to the nerve root involved. Unless all physical and neurological tests are positive for pressure symptoms, a diagnosis of a disc lesion should not be made. This condition is too important to diagnose on insufficient evidence. This has been customary in far too many low back/leg pain cases. We now have one more symptom caused by a subluxation. Known pain syndromes from anterior primary rami injury due to a subluxation are real and can now be neurologically linked.

There is one other tissue reaction that is caused by a chronic joint disrelation or subluxation that can be shown. It has been indicated how soft tissue surrounding the subluxation may shorten and become fibrotic. When this eventually occurs, the tissue will begin to calcify and progress to a traumatic degenerative change.[14] A differentiation for this entity could be an isolated arthritic joint succeeding a known chronic subluxation. In all isolated arthritic joints, a disrelation or subluxation of a chronic nature should be suspected.

Under certain circumstances, a traumatic disrelation/subluxation to a spinal motor unit is the cause of traumatic motor unit arthritis.[15] This type of arthritis is a symptom of the subluxations. To sum up the above discussion, the following are the known symptoms of a spinal subluxation/disrelation lesion.

Known Symptoms of a Subluxation/Disrelation Lesion

1. Protective muscle splinting
2. Low back pain, posterior primary rami reaction, due to joint injury and splinting
3. Known body areas of pain due to anterior and posterior primary nerve root injury and/or reaction
4. Paresthesia may occur in the more serious nerve injuries
5. Acute traumatic arthritis, all contributing to:
6. Disability due to pain, muscle contraction, and tissue changes involving the spinal motor unit

It has been shown that subluxation/disrelation of a spinal motor unit can be a primary syndrome and has symptoms that can be determined and recorded.[16] The presence of a sequel in the form of traumatic arthritis was also shown: it could present serious and lasting consequences to the patient.

It is advisable to remember that a secondary subluxation/disrelation syndrome may be present and reactive within the confines of a spinal constitutional pathology and could be the only reactive entity. The diagnosis of a pathological or traumatic subluxation/disrelation is not easy, but can be accomplished. Each symptom present in low back/leg pain must be considered on an individual basis.

In low back/leg pain cases, the patient visits the chiropractor because of pain. With each patient, the pain may vary from dull to sharp, constant to intermittent, or may be present only during certain movements. The presence of pain syndromes to the anterior or posterior primary rami can be determined and this knowledge aids in the differential diagnosis of each case. Next is an illustration of how this knowledge is advantageous.

BASIC INFORMATION FOR DIFFERENTIAL DIAGNOSIS

This knowledge immediately indicates to the physician whether or not an anterior or posterior, primary nerve root is activated. Absence of the anterior primary nerve root involvement leaves three pain areas, the paraspinal, lumbar, and gluteal syndromes. These are supplied by the posterior primary rami and are a part of or susceptible to the effects of antalgic or protective muscle contraction. This means that pain will be at the joint, near the joint, or to those muscles or both, or their attachments, or both, that are directly associated with spinal motion. By knowing the muscles of motion and the spinal levels of their nerve supply, it is possible to isolate the nerve plexus that is involved and the segmental examination further confirms the location of the reactive segment, or segments.

The presence of the anterior primary rami pain area/or areas will lead back to one of two spinal neural levels, the lumbar plexus or the sacral plexus.

Matching the findings in the following manner indicates the relationship between the pain area and the spinal nerve plexus of which the segment is a part: (This information should be included in any report to an insurance company, attorney, etc.)

Charted pain area
↓ ↑
Spinal nerve supplying that body area
↓ ↑
Same spinal nerve to spinal segment or motor unit in that nerve plexus
↓ ↑
Spinal motor unit injured and determined by the segmental examination

The differential diagnosis required to isolate the subluxation/disrelation lesion from gross spinal pathology and its various subdivisions is quite specific.

The subluxation/disrelation lesion includes a group of spinal lesions that produce abnormalities to the functioning of the spinal joint and its associated tissues. The abnormalities produced by these lesions are pain, both local or remote from the spine, antalgic muscle contraction, joint or motor unit changes, and functional changes. These changes cause a reduction of the load limit for that injured joint or motor unit that limits the ability of that spinal group to function at its maximum capacity as a unit. Each of these abnormalities can be evaluated, enabling a differential diagnosis for low back or leg pain.

The first consideration for the differential diagnosis of spinal joint or motor unit injury is to determine whether the lesion is a primary or secondary lesion. In some cases, it will only be a single joint lesion; in others, the plexus as a whole may have to be considered because of multiple joint lesions—in other words, injury to the lumbar or sacral plexus. In most cases, the history will give us valuable information. Immediate traumatic injuries to a normal spine, evaluated and found negative by x-ray, with no history of periodic back problems, even without an indication of gross pathology, would have to be evaluated as a secondary spinal lesion. All reactive spinal lesions associated with abnormal joint changes due to existing pathology, confirmed by x-ray, are secondary lesions, although they may be in an acute state from an immediate injury. All cases of low back, leg pain, or both in which the patient is unable to indicate any form of accident or abnormal stress as a contributing cause of the joint injury should be classified as a secondary lesion.

Knowledge of the precise location of the individual pain syndromes gives the next clue. This informs the chiropractor which primary neural rami is involved and enables an adequate evaluation of the mechanism of pain for that case. (Note: Without this information there is less than a 50:50 chance of formulating a correct diagnosis.) Reaction to only the posterior primary rami alerts the chiropractor that the joint or motor unit injury or changes have not extended to the nerves found in the anterior primary rami. The diagnosis of the spinal lesion with this configuration would be a facet syndrome or a subluxation/disrelation lesion, or both. If this facet syndrome is associated with a previous pathological joint, or motor unit, that condition should also be indicated in the diagnosis. Example: 2nd lumbar facet syndrome with associated osteoarthritis, or a 2nd lumbar facet syndrome associated with disc degeneration, or many other underlying pathologies, would be possible. The spinal segmental level indicated would be only that segment or segments that are found reactive during the spinal segmental examination.

(NOTE: There is an exception. The gluteal pain syndrome arises from the posterior primary rami, but causes pain away from the spine and does not appear to be directly associated with low back motion as we normally consider it. Its diagnosis should be placed in the category related to the anterior primary rami; however, to classify it as a facet syndrome would not be incorrect. It must be stated here that a facet syndrome is a named subluxation/disrelation lesion. All spinal joint lesions, named or not, that abnormally affect the spinal joint are disrelation lesions.)

Subluxation/disrelation lesions causing neural reaction to nerves found within the anterior primary rami indicates that the lesion is greater, and that its influence extends to include the nerve root and its associated tissues. Pain syndromes from this rami will then be present. Those pain syndromes from the lumbar plexus as previously mentioned will be the inguinal, Thomas, anterior femoral, and the lateral femoral. The one exception noted earlier is the gluteal syndrome. The pain syndrome from the sacral plexus will be the posterior femoral pain syndrome, which includes the posterior femoral nerve and the great sciatic nerve. The lesion level will depend upon the findings from the segmental examination.

Lesions to the anterior primary rami and their pain syndromes may be diagnosed in two ways.

1. They may be individually named, such as the gluteal pain syndrome, lateral femoral pain syndrome, inguinal pain syndrome, posterior femoral pain syndrome, etc., and the reactive lesion level (subluxation/disrelation) should be indicated for each pain syndrome area. In those cases in which a named lesion such as nerve entrapment, stenosis, or **a confirmed disc lesion is present,** confirmed by CAT or MRI, that diagnosis would also be correct.
2. If only one plexus is involved, the lumbar or sacral plexus, it may be classified as a lumbar, or sacral plexus lesion. If both are involved, then the diagnosis would be a lumbosacral plexus lesion. (The reactive spinal level [subluxation/disrelation lesion] and the pain syndrome area from each plexus should be indicated.)

(NOTE: There is an exception: The quadratus lumborum muscle is supplied by the anterior primary rami and is part of the muscle group related to spinal motion. When this muscle is activated in the form of antalgic contraction, the reactive spinal lesion or lesions should be classified as a facet syndrome. Antalgic contraction to the psoas muscle, even though it is not related to a major pain syndrome, should be considered the same. Those patients with this configuration are unable to stand erect and the direction of the body flexion indicates the muscle group involved.)

The location of pain at the back of the upper leg, from injury or reaction to the great sciatic nerve, remains the same as from injury and/or reaction to the posterior femoral nerve. **The degree of motor unit injury determines the reactive ramification of this lesion and the response from associated tissues. The type of motor**

unit injury determines which nerve would be primarily involved. The presence of multiple pain syndrome areas is directly related in most cases to the degree of spinal injury rather than the type of motor unit injury. That is, if severe enough, a posterior femoral nerve injury may mimic a disc lesion causing multiple pain syndromes although the examination findings differ. This condition then represents composite pain syndromes as described in Chapter 16, and the diagnosis must then be a lumbosacral plexus lesion. For this reason, it is essential to differentiate posterior femoral nerve lesions from a disc lesion involving the sciatic nerve.

The underlying cause of pain and its intensity may differ considerably because the subluxation/disrelation lesion includes several forms of injury or motor unit changes. Stenosis, another form of a subluxation/disrelation lesion, may be detected by x-ray, or become suspect, and the differential diagnosis between the posterior femoral syndrome and sciatica in these cases is determined by the different findings from the basic examination. The practitioner might consider a statement by Elizabeth Bradley and Philip Wood: ". . . even under the topic of low back pain there is generally insufficient differentiation between lumbago and sciatica, distinctions which the concept of disc prolapse has unhelpfully tended to blur."[17] This problem can be corrected by conducting the basic examination shown in this manual.

The most important difference for the existence of posterior femoral pain caused by a sciatic nerve lesion is that the overall injury to the motor unit is far greater, disc pressure may be present, or the greater reaction may be caused by stenosis or severe facet jamming. Inflammation and soft tissue changes at the nerve root is one cause of sciatic involvement. Another cause appears to be local antalgic contraction, restricting motion to that joint, thus producing pain, although this would probably cause posterior femoral pain rather than sciatic nerve injury. Not only will the orthopedic findings related to the 4th and/or 5th lumbar segments be positive in sciatic cases, but the spinal segmental examination to either or both those levels must show a significant reaction. Properly evaluated, these tests at the motor unit carry considerably more weight than neurologic tests to the legs, such as the pin wheel, because of the overlapping nerve supply by the posterior femoral nerve.

Even when all tests confirm sciatic neuritis and/or neuralgia, the diagnosis of a disc lesion in these cases should only be considered a possibility in the cause of pain until the presence of a disc protrusion or fragmentation is confirmed by a CAT scan or MRI. If confirmed, the lesion must be at the level of the reactive segment. Any other level, nonreactive, even with a confirmed disc lesion, should not be considered as the direct cause of pain. J. S. Lawrence indicates that disc degeneration is found in approximately 45% of the population.[18] The disc in the adult, however, does not contain nerve endings capable of registering pain. The disc may become pathological without producing symptoms. Bradley and Wood state, "Much of the literature on back complaints is confused by references to prolapse of the intervertebral disc. Although these structures undoubtedly may prolapse, herniate, or in other ways be displaced, the difficulty lies in establishing both when this may have happened, and whether it is clinically significant."[19] It is also quite appropriate that the following statement was written under the same heading regarding disc narrowing: "The result is loose usage of the term disc prolapse by both practitioner and the public, whereas the former often mislead themselves, for reasons such as we have noted, or perhaps to conceal ignorance."

Although important from an academic standpoint regarding the progression of spinal joint pathology, the **three-joint complex,** a term also mentioned in literature about spinal joint changes, should not be confused with the diagnosis of spinal joint lesions related to low back/leg pain. The term relates to the two articular facets and the disc, which are naturally related to one another; permanent injury to one will eventually affect the other. The protective mechanism of the body attempts to ensure that further neural injury is reduced by fixing and isolating this joint from the rest of the motion unit. This is done by tissue changes immediately at the injured joint but also may occur to other joints and soft tissues not at that joint.

It is the physician's responsibility to assure if possible that this permanent fixation is established with the facets in the best possible nonreactive, or reduced reactive position. Any abnormal stage of these mutual changes is a subluxation/disrelation lesion and must be diagnosed as such when they produce pain. The spinal segmental examination can determine whether a motor unit is reactive and causing pain. The history and visual signs, via x-ray, and so on, of gross pathology determine its status as a primary or secondary lesion. The finding from the basic examination, the reactive spinal segment, history, x-rays, CAT scan, and MRI, if needed, enable the physician to differentiate the type of subluxation lesion. It can then be determined if it should be classified as a subluxation/

disrelation lesion or listed under its named subclassification such as a facet syndrome, stenosis, disc lesion, hypermobile joint, hypomobile joint, and so on.

REFERENCES

1. Good AB: Spinal joint blocking. *JMPT* 8(1):1, 1985
2. Hadley LA: Intervertebral joint subluxation, bony impingement and foramen encroachment with nerve root changes. *AJR* 26(3):377, 1951
3. American Medical Association: The extremities, spine and pelvis. In *Guides to the Evaluation of Permanent Impairment* 2nd ed, Chicago, American Medical Association, 1984;p.47
4. Pressman AH, Nickles SL: Neurophysiological and nutritional consideration of pain control. *JMPT* 7(4):219, 1984
5. Farfan HF: The use of mechanical etiology to determine the efficacy of active intervention in single joint lumbar intervertebral joint problems. *Spine* 10(4): 350, 1985
6. Farfan HF: The use of mechanical etiology to determine the efficacy of active intervention in single joint lumbar intervertebral joint problems. *Spine* 10(4): 350, 1985
7. Zohn D, Mennell JM: *Diagnosis and Physical Treatment of Musculoskeletal Pain,* 3rd ed. Boston, Little, Brown & Co, 1976;p.9
8. Good AB: Spinal joint blocking. *JMPT* 8(1):1, 1985
9. Good AB: Spinal joint blocking. *JMPT* 8(1):1, 1985
10. Farfan HF: The use of mechanical etiology to determine the efficacy of active intervention in single joint lumbar intervertebral joint problems. *Spine* 10(4): 350, 1985
11. Gray H: *Gray's Anatomy,* 30th ed. Philadelphia, Lea & Febiger, 1984;p.1223
12. Hoppenfeld S: *Orthopedic Neurology*. Philadelphia, JB Lippincott, 1977;p.67
13. Rydevik B, Mark B, Lundborg G: Pathoanatomy and pathophysiology of nerve root compression. *Spine* 9(1): 7, 1984
14. Farfan HF: The use of mechanical etiology to determine the efficacy of active intervention in single joint lumbar intervertebral joint problems. *Spine* 10(4): 350, 1985
15. Farfan HF: The use of mechanical etiology to determine the efficacy of active intervention in single joint lumbar intervertebral joint problems. *Spine* 10(4): 350, 1985
16. Kirkaldy-Willis WH: The relationship of structural pathology to the nerve root. *Spine* 9(1):49, 1984
17. Bradley E, Wood P: *The Lumbar Spine and Back Pain,* 3rd ed. New York, Churchill Livingstone, 1987;p.7
18. Lawrence JS: Disc degeneration. *Ann Rheum Dis* 28:121, 1969

Chapter 5

The Mechanism of Low Back/Leg Pain

*I*nformation from this chapter will be found and referred to throughout the chapters of this book. The low back, pelvic, and leg pain syndromes with their causative agent, the spinal lesion, are a part of the complex neural system that the chiropractor must deal with on a daily basis. It is vital to know how spinal injuries affect tissues at the joint and also how these injuries may create reactive responses through the nervous system to other areas of the spine and/or away from the spine. The evaluation of spinal injuries, with their pain syndromes, depends upon the practitioner's ability to conduct a differential diagnostic procedure and, once evaluated, how the findings relate to one another within the mechanism of pain. A positive or negative test in low back/leg pain cases is of little or no value until the physician is cognizant of the neural components, and has a working knowledge of their reactions. The physician must also recognize that the existence of gross spinal pathology is not a requisite for low back, pelvic, and leg pain syndromes.

All attempts to correlate the various forms of spinal pathology to low back/leg pain have failed. Spinal pathologies such as constitutional disease of bone, birth defect, curvatures, and so on, often produce little or no pain to the spinal joint or joints involved. Even injuries to the low back do not readily reveal the spinal segment or segments injured. Present day nonviable examination procedures fail to produce consistent findings to relate the pain areas suffered by the patient to his/her physical manifestations.[1] The result of this failure is that different physicians examining the same patient often arrive at diverse conclusions. Because treatment is based upon these conclusions, this treatment also varies and may not be in the best interest of the patient.

The key to a greater understanding of low back/leg pain must emerge from increased knowledge of the pain areas and their characteristics. Also necessary is the understanding of the responses or findings deduced from the regional orthopedic examination, and the reaction from an examination of each spinal segment that might be involved. These examination procedures for low back/leg pain cases **must be consistent, and must be conducted in every case of low back/leg pain,** in order to become familiar with variations in patient response and subtle differences in tissue reaction.[2]

The knowledge and understanding of spinal pathology is essential; yet, years of research in low-back pathology have not brought either the chiropractic or medical physician closer to understanding pain caused by injuries to the lower spinal segments. We now know that pain as a subjective symptom can be outlined and recorded, thus creating the eight constant low back, pelvic, and leg pain syndromes.[3] The precise examination of each spinal segment and the findings provide additional information in the determination of those tissues involved in low back/leg pain cases. The investigation of neuroanatomy, associated with the pain syndromes and spinal segmental findings, has shown that low back, pelvic, and leg pain syndromes are not confined to injury of only one spinal area, but may arise from the 10th thoracic to the 5th lumbar, or any combination of those.

RECORDED FINDINGS FOR LOW BACK/LEG PAIN CASES

The examination of thousands of individual spinal segments has shown that two spinal regions appear to be injured or reactive most frequently, the thoracolumbar and the lumbosacral.[4] The examination has also shown that the thoracolumbar region is injured or reactive precisely twice as frequently as the lumbosacral region.[5] As these two anatomical and neural levels are evaluated, we find that pain syndromes are also divided between these two levels. They are the lumbar plexus associated with the thoracolumbar anatomical region, and the sacral plexus associated with the 4th lumbar and lumbosacral joint. Each plexus is also divided into two main neural systems: firstly, the posterior primary rami, and secondly, the anterior primary rami, each neural system causing specific pain syndromes.

The posterior primary rami are responsible for

31

the paraspinal, lumbar, and gluteal syndromes.[6] The anterior primary rami are responsible for the Thomas, inguinal, anterior femoral, lateral femoral, and posterior femoral syndromes. A 5th lumbar disc lesion causing sciatica (not a primary pain syndrome) involves the anterior primary rami of the sacral plexus. When any or all three pain syndromes mentioned (associated with the posterior primary rami) are activated in the presence of a sciatic or leg pain case, we can include involvement of the lumbar plexus level. Spinal segmental reaction of lumbar plexus levels also indicates reaction of the lumbar plexus posterior primary rami and may be present in the absence of lumbar plexus pain syndromes because this reaction may not be severe enough to activate those pain syndromes. This information enables the chiropractor to better evaluate the kind and level of treatment necessary for known pain syndromes. These levels can be easily determined by a working knowledge of the pain syndromes and the tissues that are reactive due to overstimulation.

Pain Mechanism
Due to the unusual finding of the two major spinal levels of reaction from the spinal segments, an investigation of this mechanism was conducted. The following gives an account of the information obtained.

1. The spinal neural system is capable of reaction to the injury of any of its components by an antalgic protective mechanism. This mechanism can bring into play any portion of the nervous system, regardless of its physiological or anatomical location, when needed for protection. Its influence extends to any body tissue that might be required for its protection.
2. This mechanism can produce a lesion of the spine, or outside the spinal area, if required, to prevent or reduce a greater lesion.
3. The body appears to adjust the spinal muscular system to a general load level compatible with the spine's weakest joint.[7]

In order to understand the mechanism, this author's work when combined with the work of others leads to this conclusion that the body's response to injury or pain is some form of reaction. This reaction is protective, a splinting of the spinal segments as an aid to prevent further injury. Injury to spinal joints activates the posterior primary rami at that level. Deep muscles surrounding the joint contract, causing antalgic splinting. During the acute or reactive stage, this status is picked up by the segmental examination. If the condition becomes chronic, soft tissue changes and its ability to respond in a normal fashion is impaired; it may become dormant until another injury reactivates it. During the dormant stage, the patient may be relatively pain free. It appears, however, that the dormant stage is not taken lightly by the nervous system. Excess neural impulses from soft tissue damage may continue and thus activate the anterior primary rami, causing pain syndromes from that division.[8-12]

This mechanism appears to react in a manner shown in Figure 5–1. (Note: posterior primary rami firing from a low-grade lesion affects the anterior primary rami. Those rami causing muscle response with associated pain are shown in Figures 5–2 and 5–3.

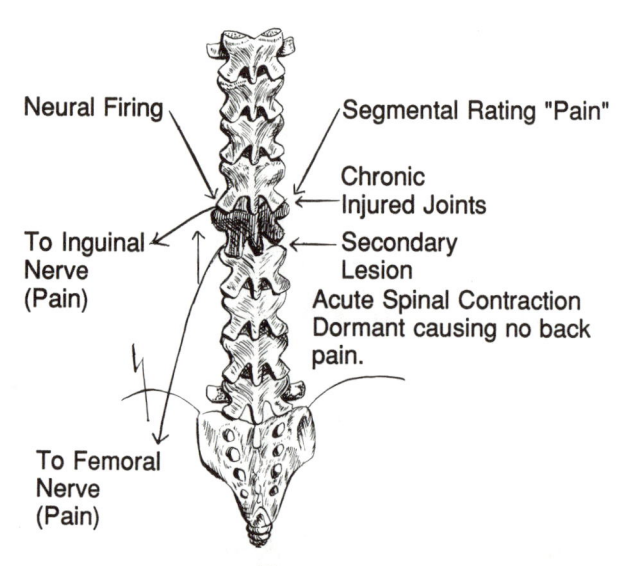

Figure 5–1

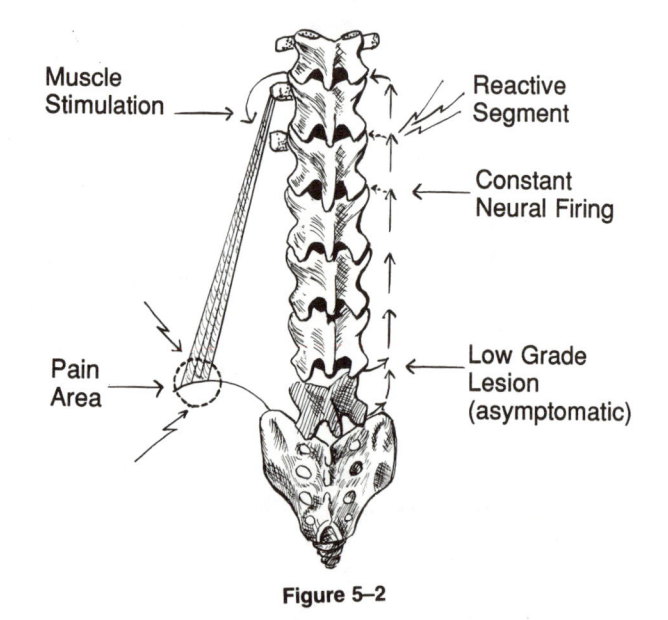

Figure 5–2

A lesion at the 5th lumbar may initiate a neural reaction to the posterior primary neural rami, causing muscle contraction only at that level. Should the injury or reaction be greater, the local deep muscles may not offer enough protection, and the demand for greater protection would have to activate the lumbar posterior primary nerve division. This division supplies the major muscles of the low back, with some exceptions. The quadratus lumborum is supplied by the anterior primary rami. In severe cases, this portion of the anterior primary rami may also be activated, causing the patient to bend toward the side of contraction when this muscle is activated (see Fig. 5–3).

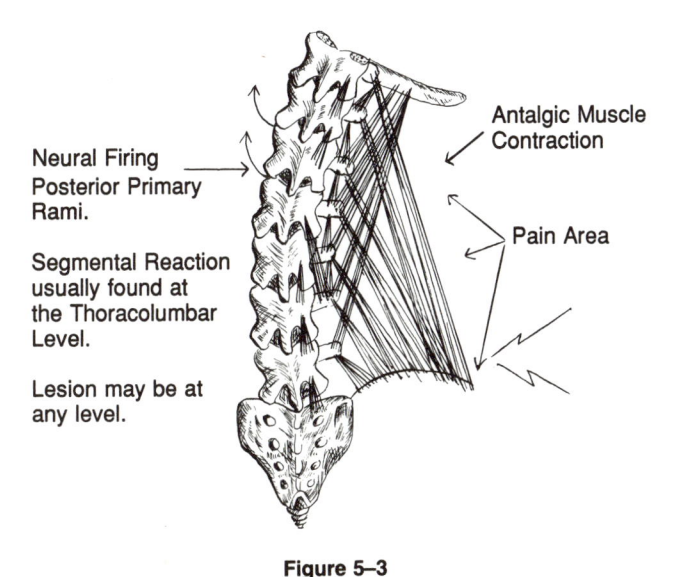

The psoas muscle may also contract in varying degrees, flexing the body in a protective mechanism for the injured or reactive spinal joints. Moreover, further investigation has shown that lumbosacral pain, thought to be caused by injury to that joint, is in fact more often caused by injury to, or reaction from, the supraspinal ligament. Severe debilitating pain can be caused by injury to or reaction from the supraspinal ligament without reaction from the lumbosacral joint. An interesting observation arises as to the possible cause of supraspinal ligament pain because it does not always relate to lumbosacral injury. It appears to be related to thoracolumbar injury: specific spinal manipulation of the thoracolumbar region has a beneficial effect upon the supraspinal ligament pain. Almost every case has responded to that form of treatment in a highly satisfactory manner. Those few that did not respond as well have x-ray evidence of gross spinal pathology at the thoracolumbar level. It may well be possible that this phenomenon could be one cause of both failed spinal surgery at the lumbosacral joint and failure when conservative treatment is given only to the lumbosacral joint (see Fig. 5–4).

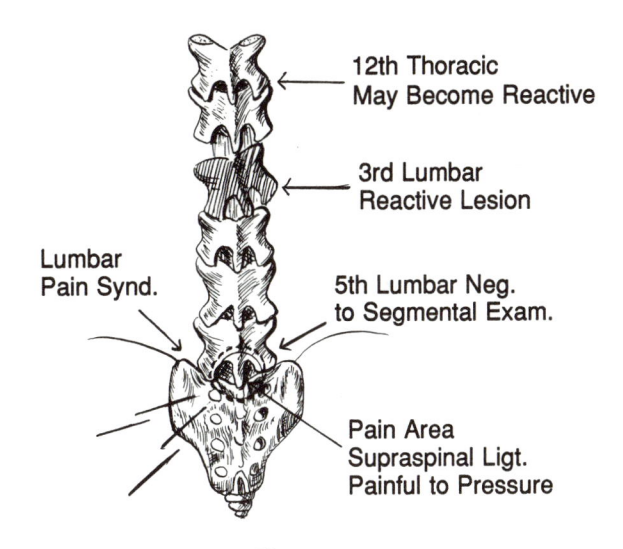

Figure 5–3

Figure 5–4

If investigation of the nerve supply to the low back muscles including the quadratus lumborum and psoas muscles is conducted, it will be found that their major nerve supply arises from the 10th thoracic to the 3rd lumbar spinal motor units, thus placing them in the thoracolumbar region. Reaction at the 12th thoracic motor unit far surpasses the combined count of all other spinal segments involving low back/leg pain syndromes.

It appears that injury in any form to the lumbar spinal motor units can cause mild to severe reaction at the 12th thoracic/1st lumbar neural level, resulting in variations in the protective mechanism. Because the greatest number of pain syndromes is produced from the 12th thoracic to the 2nd lumbar motor unit, we cannot ignore the fact that injuries may be more frequent to that level than is generally considered. All the cases that react at the thoracolumbar region do not, however, appear to be caused by local injury. When reaction occurs at the thoracolumbar region, more specifically the 12th thoracic/1st lumbar nerves (12th thoracic, iliohypogastric, ilioinguinal, and 1st lumbar nerve), permanent injury may be caused from this neural response, particularly if treatment is delayed. Studies of this region over a period of many years with associated syndromes have left no doubt that permanent injury and/or impairment can and does occur. It appears that once a static position at the spinal motor unit is produced regardless of the cause, with injury at the joint, or joint reaction as a protective mechanism, soft tissue changes become the sequel with resulting pathological changes and susceptibility to lumbar plexus pain syndromes.[13,14] These joint changes are a subluxation of a second degree. It also appears that pathological changes can occur to muscle attachments to bone in the form of fibrosis when consistent contraction of that muscle or muscle fibers is present. This change may be the cause of many chronic pain areas close to bone (see Figures 5-5, and 5-6).

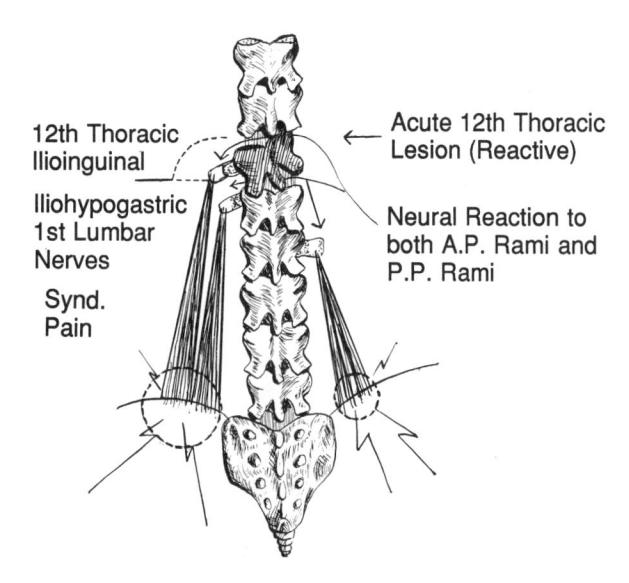

Figure 5-5

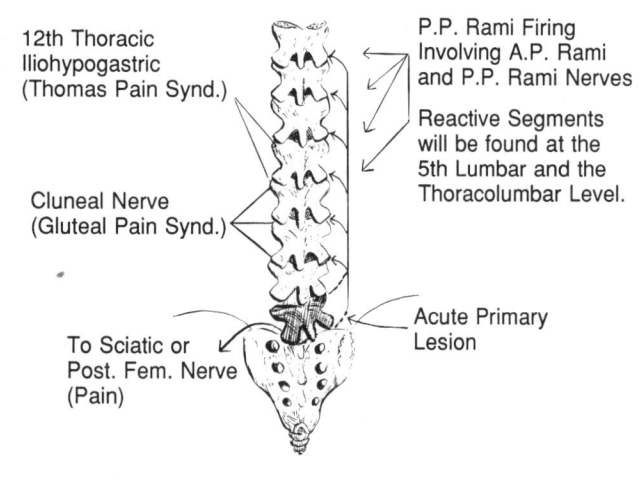

Figure 5-6

CONCLUSION

In order to diagnose and treat low back/leg pain on a more efficient level than is being done today, a better understanding of pain syndromes is necessary, including their perimeters, frequency, association, nerve supplies, and spinal levels involved. Laboratory researchers cannot be faulted in their quest for more information regarding gross and microscopic pathology of the spinal motor unit, but clinical research is a must, and an ever-important midway point between the patient who suffers low back/leg pain and the researcher for spinal pathology. Facts can be obtained in general office practice that may be obscure to the laboratory researcher. Clinical observation with statistical background can be a stepping stone that increases our understanding of the neurological responses of the body to spinal motor unit injury, regardless of the cause.

REFERENCES

1. Mooney V: Problems in compensation systems promote employee back disability. *Back Pain Monitor* 2:16, 1984
2. Thomas JE: Classification of low back/leg pain syndromes, Part 3. *FCA Journal* January–February:37, 1986
3. Thomas JE: Classification of low back/leg pain syndromes, Part 2. *FCA Journal* November–December: 18, 1985
4. Thomas JE: Classification of low back/leg pain syndromes, Part 4. *FCA Journal* July–August:32, 1986
5. Hoppenfeld S: *Orthopedic Neurology.* Philadelphia, JB Lippincott, 1977;p.98
6. Hamilton WJ: *Textbook of Human Anatomy,* 2nd ed. St. Louis MO: C.V. Mosby Co, 1976;p.638
7. Gracovitsky S, Farfan H: The optimum spine. *Spine* 11(6):543, 1986
8. Gray H: *Gray's Anatomy.* Philadelphia, Lea & Febiger, 1984;p.464
9. Wood L: Acute locked facet syndrome and its treatment by manipulation under local periarticular anesthesia—Part 1: Clinical perspective and pilot study proposal. *JMPT* 7(4):211, 1984
10. Gray H: *Gray's Anatomy.* Philadelphia, Lea & Febiger, 1984;p.1198
11. Hamilton WJ: *Textbook of Human Anatomy,* 2nd ed. St. Louis MO, C.V. Mosby Co, 1976;p.138
12. Gray H: *Gray's Anatomy.* Philadelphia, Lea & Febiger, 1984;p.464
13. Wood L: Acute locked facet syndrome and its treatment by manipulation under local periarticular anesthesia—Part 1: Clinical perspective and pilot study proposal. *JMPT* 7(4):211, 1984
14. Pressman AH, Nickles SL: Neurophysiological and nutritional consideration of pain control. *JMPT* 7(4):219, 1984

Chapter 6

Regional Orthopedic Examination for Low Back/Leg Pain

The examination of each low back case is as important as the examination of any other disease process from which the patient might suffer. Low back/leg pain is a condition suffered by millions of people, causing untold loss of labor hours at a staggering cost; thus, its importance is a priority in all of its facets. It is stated quite well by W.H. Kirkaldy-Willis.[1] The author contends that there is no place in the management of low back pain for any approach other than one that begins by using the most precise and scientific methods available.

There are many tests and procedures shown in a variety of texts that are available for use within a basic examination procedure, but few have the value required when used in the examination of **all cases of low back, pelvic, and leg pain.** Any procedure used in these cases should give a reasonably specific answer for all cases regarding the status of the tissue being investigated. In low back, pelvic, and leg pain cases any reaction from the joint, nerve root, disc, and various associated muscles must be considered in order to arrive at a correct diagnosis.

There are tests such as motion studies, spinal percussion, buckling sign, Sicard's test, Turyn's test, bowstring sign, Kemp sign, and the Dejerine's Triad, as well as neurological tests to the legs. Also, some tests are available to aid in determining a pathological hip or a sacroiliac joint lesion. The findings from these tests either overlap tests found in the basic examination as shown in this manual, or are those that may be useful under certain conditions in addition to and following the basic tests. The Kemp sign and Dejerine's Triad are excellent tests for sciatic involvement and the possibilities of a disc lesion to either the cervical or lumbar region. If, however, an anterior primary rami nerve is not involved in a case producing symptoms, these tests are unnecessary and do not, therefore, contribute to the basic procedure. Motion studies are an indicator of the ability or inability of the patient to perform normal movements. They do not indicate the level of a spinal lesion causing disability when present, nor do they indicate whether gross or nongross pathology exists. Furthermore, motion studies do not indicate that all segments within that region are functioning. Without information from the basic examination it is not apparent that the problem arises from pathological changes away from the spine. It is of little value to conduct a neurologic examination of the legs when it is obvious that the anterior primary rami supplying one or more nerves to the legs is not involved. Spinal segmental lesions causing pain must be eliminated before sacroiliac and hip lesions are considered, unless those lesions are so obvious that they require immediate attention. Hence, even without the basic examination, the diagnosis might be inaccurate. The tests mentioned should be used when needed for possible added clarification, but more importantly to evaluate the degree of injury once the reactive joint is determined, and even then only considered for their evaluation within the total examination procedure.

This chapter and Chapter 7 outline precise procedures for the low back, pelvic, and leg pain examination that if followed with care will give an effective working tool for the differential diagnosis of low back/leg pain.

EXAMINATION PROCEDURES

Immediately after the initial history is taken and a general visual inspection of the patient is conducted, the physician asks for a description of the area of pain.

Direct the patient to outline the area of pain with his or her fingertips over each area of pain, if more than one exists. This should be done in every case regardless of the practitioner's familiarity with an area suggested by the patient. (Example: The patient might state that the abdomen is painful and point to the groin; most commonly, he or she may state that the hip is painful and point to the gluteal muscles.) It is important that the patient is specific in pointing out the area of pain. Each area of pain should be recorded as it is indicated.

When determined, the areas of pain should be drawn on figures found on most case history cards. This provides a permanent visual picture of the pain area. The name of each syndrome should also be recorded on each card, providing a word picture useful in discussing the case with other physicians, attorneys, insurance companies, and the patient. For example, if the patient has a paraspinal syndrome, that diagnosis can be stated with the confidence that a simple description is available. Once the pain areas are recorded and named, the patient is readied for the examination.

Men should strip to the waist with belts and buttons loosened. Gowns that open at the back should be given to women, with instructions to remove all clothing except loose underpants.

The examination of the patient should be conducted in a room containing a physiotherapy or examination table; chiropractic treatment tables are not practical for this purpose. The best examination tables are no less than 22 inches wide. An even wider table gives the patient added security from the fear of falling. **Do not conduct any other examination until the following examinations are completed.**

This examination should be completed on all patients suffering from low back, pelvic, or leg pain, regardless of the area of pain. The same routine is conducted for a paraspinal pain syndrome as for an anterior femoral pain syndrome, and so on. No part of the examination should ever be omitted. It is essential that negative findings also be recorded, as these are, in the final analysis, as important as the positive findings.

First, the 12th thoracic and 4th lumbar segments are located and marked as shown in Figure 6–1. The examination should be conducted as follows.

Straight Leg Raising (SLR) Test

In order to understand the SLR test the physician must first determine what is being looked for and what findings are anticipated when conducting this phase of the orthopedic examination.

There are two basic low back spinal areas that can be involved with an injury or spinal lesion. These two areas respond to injury or pathology in slightly different ways. The purpose of the SLR test is to give an indication of which area is reactive, or if both are reactive. This is accomplished by an understanding of the tissues that respond to this

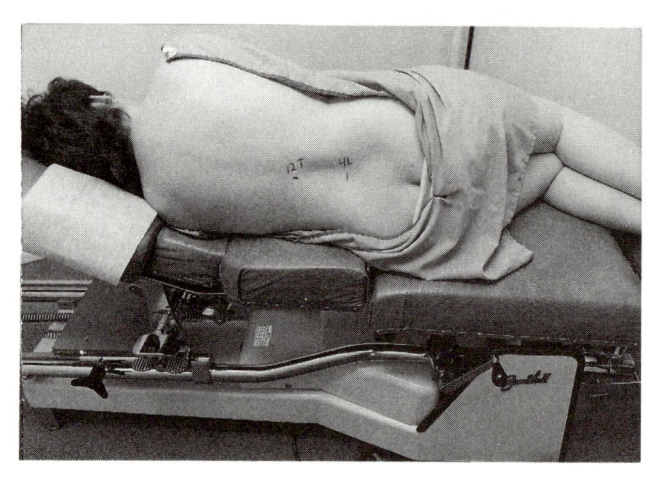

Figure 6–1

test from each spinal area, and the manner in which they react.

The two anatomical areas are the lumbar plexus and the sacral plexus; their associated nerve groups supply certain specific pain syndromes, thus causing different tissues to react. The areas of the pain syndromes have already been determined before this test is initiated. This information gives advance knowledge as to the possible area involved.

We are looking for negative or positive reactive findings from tissues related to each of the plexus areas. Because the lumbosacral joint is moved during this test, it is the major tissue tested in the determination of sacral plexus lesions. The tilting of the pelvis during this test also places stress upon low back muscles and attachments that are neurologically supplied by nerves from the lumbar plexus. The test aids in this differentiation. When positive findings are discovered, the tissue area must be stated, followed by the reactive rating. The rating would be

1. Mild
2. Medium
3. Sharp or severe

Example:

- Lumbosacral joint. Neg. (this indicates no reaction)
- Lumbosacral joint. Pos. mild (reactive finding)
- Iliac crest (center) Pos. medium
- Iliac crest (lateral) Pos. sharp
- Iliac crest (medial) Pos. mild
- Gluteal Pos. sharp
- R. leg (posterior) sharp
- Inguinal (groin–center) Pos. sharp

With the patient in a supine position, head resting on a medium-hard pillow, a bilateral straight-leg raising test is conducted. The patient is instructed not to assist in raising the legs. The leg is not raised beyond 90°, and it must be raised fairly slowly to allow the patient time to accurately determine the area of pain if it is present.

Pain to the Back of the Leg

As the leg is raised, the first consideration is pain at or in the back of the leg. If the patient does not indicate a posterior femoral/sciatic pain syndrome, it is possible that some pain may be produced from tight leg muscles or other disease processes at the knee that are not associated with spinal pathology. This will be found primarily in the older patient. If the patient has a posterior femoral pain syndrome, some pain may be present at the upper leg. The presence of sciatic pain is usually severe, and the test will increase this pain. The patient will indicate the pain and resist further leg raising. The pain should be gauged and the leg raised further *if possible*. It serves no purpose to raise the leg too vigorously if sharp pain is present. If the patient with recorded posterior leg pain experiences increased pain as the leg is raised, the leg should be lowered until the increased pain is absent. At this position, the ankle should be flexed; if a severe increase in leg pain is not indicated, the sciatic nerve is probably not involved. A sharp increase in pain at the back of the leg will usually indicate possible sciatic nerve involvement; if dull or less painful, it probably arises from deeper pain centers in the muscle, from the posterior femoral nerve, or from both. When no posterior leg pain is indicated, or if present is not too severe, the physician continues to raise the leg; the pelvis will begin to lift or flex toward the abdomen. The presence of a gluteal or Thomas syndrome may cause pain in those areas. When either the gluteal or the posterior portion of the Thomas syndrome is present, the pain may or may not be increased by the SLR test. If the pain from these syndromes is cutaneous, little increase will be noted. A chronic syndrome that might involve underlying tissues will probably cause an increase in pain. This is particularly true in the gluteal syndrome. Underlying muscle contraction in the gluteal region could cause a sharp increase in pain over both the gluteal region and the posterior portion of the Thomas syndrome. This is apt to occur only when lower lumbar nerves are involved, and could occur with or without the gluteal syndrome. When no increase in pain is caused by the SLR test, but the presence of pain syndromes exists, we cannot classify the patient as pain-free, but that the test is negative. At about this same level of straight leg raising, pain may be noted at the lumbosacral joint or along the crests of the ilium. When no pain is noted, the physician continues to raise the leg to the full 90° for verification that this test is negative.

The existence of lumbosacral pain and iliac crest pain are two separate reactions arising from the two different areas, and must be discussed separately.

Pain at the Lumbosacral Joint

The lumbar syndrome is a small pain area located directly over the lumbar vertebrae or lumbosacral joint. Straight leg raising tests for this pain syndrome appear to be inconsistent, but the reactions are, in fact, quite reliable. Pain may be caused or increased during this test, or completely absent. The reason for these variations has caused considerable consternation and probably inadequate diagnosis for many years. There are two primary causes of lumbosacral pain resulting from the SLR test. A third less common cause will also be found.

1. Injury or pathology to the motor unit
   Trauma to the lumbosacral joint will cause tissue reaction, pain, and a positive SLR test. Pathological conditions produce pain only when a tissue-reactive state exists. During a dormant period, pain is not produced. During the nonreactive state, the SLR test will be negative. If negative, the sacral plexus and associated spinal level should not be considered as a primary cause of low back/leg pain. This proves true even when the lumbar pain syndrome is present.
2. Interspinous and supraspinous ligaments
   A most prevalent cause of pain at the lumbosacral joint during the SLR test is irritation of the supraspinal ligament or its attachments. This condition often occurs without injury or reaction to the 4th or 5th lumbar joints or nerves. The existence of this pain reaction has caused innumerable incorrect diagnoses and unnecessary follow-up primary treatment to the 4th and 5th lumbar segments.[2] (Note: the spinal segmental test must be given to confirm the diagnosis, as described in Chapter 7.)
3. A neurological link between the sacral and lumbar plexuses, the third cause of lumbosacral pain, is much more complex than the first two and has been discussed in the previous chapter.[3] Finally, positive lumbosacral pain is only considered if the pain experienced by the patient is at the center line, with a maximum extension of 1½ inches extending to either side of the center line. If any doubt exists in the doctor's mind as to the exact location of pain, the patient should place his or her finger tips at the pain area during the test as soon as it is produced. As little as ½-inch

error in the location of this pain point can lead to an incorrect diagnosis.

Pain at Back Areas Other Than the Lumbosacral Joint

To continue this description of the SLR test, having recorded the previous finding, the next activity is to note the pain from slightly lateral to the 5th lumbar facets, extending along the iliac crest to the lateral midline of the body. Pain may be produced at any point along this base line. It may extend as much as 2 inches below the base line and above the base line as high as the 11th and 12th thoracic vertebrae.

A negative finding at the areas indicated simply means the defense mechanism is not strong enough to cause the muscle attachment to be painful. This holds true even if a paraspinal pain syndrome is present. Patients with lumbar and/or paraspinal pain syndromes frequently respond with a negative SLR test. **This does not indicate they are pain free. It does show that the muscles and attachments tested by this test are not under tension sufficient to produce pain.** Neither does it indicate that a psychosomatic condition is present and that they should be sent to the nearest psychiatrist.

A positive finding: Pain produced anywhere in the paraspinal triangle is an indication that the protective mechanism is reactive in this patient. If a paraspinal pain syndrome is present and pain is increased by straight leg raising, the same holds true. *(All findings must be recorded.)*

Fabere Test

Fabere (Patrick) test is used for examination of the hip (flexion, abduction, external rotation, and extension). In the United States this test is known as the Patrick sign; I prefer the name Fabere because it indicates the motions required for the test. This test has been used primarily to determine hip pathology, specifically arthritis. Expanding the use of this test to include low back, hip, groin, and leg pain enables the chiropractor to evaluate a larger area. The procedure for the Fabere test follows.

The patient's leg is flexed and the ankle placed on the opposite knee. One hand is used to gently abduct the flexed leg while the other hand exerts slight pressure on the opposite hip to prevent lifting of the pelvis.

While conducting this test, it is appropriate to keep in mind that there are three pain syndromes found in the pelvic region. The inguinal and triangular portion of the Thomas syndrome will be examined by the Fabere test. The gluteal syndrome and posterior portion of the Thomas syndrome will be examined by the SLR test.

As testing proceeds, the first consideration must be the hip joint. If deep pain or restriction of motion is noticed, arthritis or other hip pathology might be present, and further examination by x-rays would be necessary. The physician must always be aware that nonreactive arthritis or degeneration may be present in old injury or geriatric cases.

When the inguinal syndrome is present, a slight pain finding indicates surface pain. Sharp pain at the groin or iliohypogastric region in the presence or absence of the inguinal syndrome indicates local nerve hypersensitivity or underlying swelling and irritation to deeper soft tissue (lymphatics, muscle attachments, fibrotic areas, etc.).

It is not surprising that the patient experiences leg pain during the Fabere test. If the patient has a preexisting femoral syndrome, the Fabere test will probably produce pain at the anterior, medial, or lateral thigh. Irritation to the genitofemoral nerve may produce pain during the test without a preexisting femoral syndrome.[4]

Examination of the hip and adjacent tissue is complicated. When the Fabere test does not increase or produce pain, with or without the existence of the Thomas syndrome, the test is negative. This does not indicate the patient is pain free, it simply tells us the muscles and deeper tissues are not involved. The patient may have nonreactive arthritis and still produce a negative Fabere test.

When Thomas syndrome is not indicated and the test is positive, hip arthritis or other pathology should be suspected and further measures taken. This might occur in a small percentage of the cases.

The presence of the Thomas syndrome does not indicate hip pathology. It may be present over a nonreactive arthritis or a normal hip joint. Using hip pain as an indicator for joint pathology in the absence of further investigation, amounts to medical neglect. *The Thomas syndrome is supplied by the 12th thoracic nerve and radiates to the greater trochanter of the hip.*[4] The description of pain syndromes notes that the Thomas syndrome has two sections. One section is a triangle immediately above the trochanter of the femur; the other area extends over the gluteal muscle from the lateral midline of the pelvis. The portion over the gluteal muscle is usually discovered during a SLR test. The triangular portion is tested by the Fabere test and is frequently painful during the procedure. The area of pain is usually quite precise, centering slightly above the greater trochanter, and is about the size of a quarter.

One final observation to be noted: the Fabere

test may aid in the verification of the paraspinal syndrome because it often induces pain at the iliac crest. This may occur on either side. *(All findings must be recorded.)*

Soto Hall Test—Linder's Sign

Both these tests have a common basis, the ability to stretch posterior and paraspinal soft tissue of the spine with some degree of control.[5] This ability aids in localizing the spinal level involved, and allows us another indicator for that level.

The procedure used for this test is easy and quick. The patient is not permitted to assist by lifting the head or body. All movements must be performed by the chiropractor. Placing one hand below the head to support the neck, the other hand on the chest below the clavicle, the head is lifted, and the neck flexed while applying slight pressure on the chest to stabilize the trunk and shoulders. It is mandatory that the exact location if any pain produced in the lower back is observed. The reference to low back with this test includes an area from the 8th thoracic to the 5th lumbar. Most frequently, when pain is produced by this portion of the test it will be centered over the spine and fairly localized. Experience has shown that low back pain produced by this test indicates an injured spinal motor unit or a highly sensitive nerve root.[6] When this reaction is present, and the second portion of the test increases the pain, the physician should not attempt to complete the test. Should the Soto Hall test be negative, one may then proceed to the Linder's sign.

The entire examination is a test to determine nerve irritation, muscle tension, or limited motion in a variety of directions. The combination provides a picture that is necessary for the diagnosis.

The Linder's portion of this test is conducted by removing the hand that was placed on the chest and, using the hand that is behind the head and neck, gently lifting the patient's upper body from the table toward a flexed or sitting position.

Sixty or seventy degrees is ordinarily sufficient for this part of the test, but the patient should be brought to a full sitting position. If a negative finding is evident, the test is complete. A positive finding may be as follows.

As the patient's upper body is being gently flexed, pain may be produced at the lower back. (Note: If the patient is lifted too rapidly, pain can be severe and certainly would obscure differential findings.) Pain may be produced over or lateral to the spine from the 8th thoracic to the lumbosacral joint over the crest of the ilium, either unilaterally or bilaterally. The topmost spinal pain must be marked as well as the lateral spread over the iliac crest. This traces the triangle of paraspinal muscles involved. If pain is caused immediately over the lumbosacral joint, this area should be marked also. *(All findings must be recorded.)*

Conclusion of Supine Position

All routine testing for the supine position is now completed. When the inguinal and/or anterior femoral syndromes are present, or if pain was produced in these areas by the examination, additional investigation is required. The patient is asked to lie down again in a supine position, and by careful manual and visual inspection, the chiropractor eliminates or confirms the presence of contusions, swelling, fibrotic areas, vascular irregularities, or any other visible or palpable abnormalities. If any exist, they are recorded, and will then become a factor in the ultimate conclusion related to treatment, prognosis, disability, etc., for that patient. It is at this time that underlying muscles and soft tissue are gently probed to determine the depth of pain reaction. Careful probing is often more informative than a multitude of tests. When this examination is complete, the patient should rise to a sitting position with his or her legs hanging over the table.

(Never change charted pain syndromes, although pain areas may be found during palpations outside the boundaries of that pain syndrome.)

Sitting—Straight Leg Raising (SSRL)

The first SLR test was done with the patient lying down in as relaxed a position as possible, and all motion was controlled by the chiropractor.

The SSRL test requires muscular effort and spinal coordination by the patient while lifting the legs.[7]

A negative test is indicated if the patient is able to sit erect and comfortably with hands resting on the lap and can straighten each leg independently, or both together, without pain.

It is advisable to remember that when the term *negative* is used, all tests given for low back/leg pain one means that *absolutely no pain or distress* exists. There is no compromise for this finding. If the patient states, "Doctor, that's uncomfortable," or "It hurts a little," the findings cannot be recorded as negative.

Because both supine and sitting straight leg raising are testing the same areas of the body, a duplication of the results might be expected, and this does happen. When duplication occurs, the findings for that case are reenforced. It is not surprising, however, that a negative finding in the supine position becomes positive in the sitting position. In the sitting position, we are testing the patient under conditions that create slightly greater stress. The supine position is a passive test, whereas the sitting position is active.

This completes the regional orthopedic examination for low back/leg pain cases. The second portion, called the spinal segmental examination, immediately follows this examination. *(All findings must be recorded.)*

The examination forms, #110 and #111, found in the appendices at the back of this book should be used for recording low back/leg pain. They then become a permanent record for the doctor, insurance company, attorney, and so on. It also provides an accurate record for progress reports when repeated at a later date.

REFERENCES

Straight Leg Raising Test

1. Kirkaldy-Willis WH: Introduction: A scientific approach. In *Managing Low Back Pain,* 2nd ed. New York, Churchill Livingstone, 1988;p.93
2. Cox JM. *Low Back Pain,* 4th ed. Baltimore, Williams & Wilkins, 1985;p.28
3. Gray H. Fascae and muscles of the trunk. *Gray's Anatomy*. Philadelphia, Lea & Febiger, 1984;p.464

Fabere Test

4. Gray H: *Gray's Anatomy,* 30th ed. Philadelphia, Lea & Febiger, 1984;p.1229

Soto Hall Test—Linder's Sign

5. Cox JM: *Low Back Pain,* 4th ed. Baltimore, Williams & Wilkins, 1985;p.90
6. Cox JM: *Low Back Pain,* 4th ed. Baltimore, Williams & Wilkins, 1985;p.90

Sitting—Straight Leg Raising

7. Cox JM: *Low Back Pain,* 4th ed. Baltimore, Williams & Wilkins, 1985;p.100

Chapter 7

Spinal Segmental Examination

VERTEBRAL TESTING

The most complicated structure of the body is the spine. It combines bone, muscles, ligaments, blood vessels, discs, fatty tissue, and nerves into a working functional unit. This unit houses the spinal cord and enables us to move the body into complicated positions for work, fun, and self-protection.

The examination of this complex unit is a physical diagnostic procedure that was developed near the turn of the century and is still employed by present-day physicians.[1] Little has been done to update this procedure, although x-ray evidence in 1951 proved that a spinal subluxation does exist and can adversely affect nerve roots.[2]

Demands by government health programs, worker's compensation, the insurance industry, attorneys, etc., for objective signs or acceptable proof of disability caused by low back/leg pain are increasing. If these demands are not recognized and addressed by all physicians, these agents will place restrictions and limitations on spinal nerve problems that will be devastating to the patient. Some limitations now exist.

The following test is effective and accurate and should be a permanent part of all spinal examinations, particularly those cases of low back/leg pain. The procedure is presented in the text that follows:

Body Position for a Segmental Examination

The patient lies in a prone position, arms resting at his or her side or flexed over the head. If the back hurts in this position, a 4- to 6-inch-thick pillow is placed beneath the ankles and usually provides comfort to the patient.

The first step is to mark, with a skin pencil, the 4th lumbar spinous process and then count upward and mark the 12th thoracic process.

A word of caution: although the chiropractor conducts a comprehensive regional low back examination, it is vital that the level of spinal involvement is not prejudged at this time.

Examination for Spinal Segmental Reaction

The first act in examination of the low back for vertebral testing is to place one's thumb below the 5th lumbar spinous at the base of the sacrum. Pressing and sliding toward the 5th lumbar spinous, 4 to 6 pounds of pressure is applied; thus checking the supraspinal ligament. If the ligament is normal, this pressure will not produce pain.

(Note: The amount of pressure indicated has been used on several hundred patients of all ages and body textures.[3] On a thin elderly patient, less pressure is advisable. In order to gain accuracy and consistency in pressure technique, practice with a fishing scale is strongly recommended until constant pressure within the 4- to 6-pound range can be maintained. The physician should ensure that the first attempt to examine spinal segments is accurate, as repeated probing can irritate even normal tissue.)

A negative finding eliminates the probability of injury or pain to the ligaments at the lumbosacral junction. A positive reaction, pain from the 4- to 6-pounds of pressure, indicates that the supraspinal ligament has either been injured or is reactive because of joint changes to one or more of the segments above. Negative or positive, the findings from the supraspinal ligament must be kept separate from the finding indicated at the lumbosacral joint. The reason for this will be understood as discussion of joint segmental tests continues.

The next step is to evaluate pain found at each spinal level from the 5th lumbar to the 10th thoracic segment. The patient is told that an equal pressure will be applied to each vertebra during this examination, and that he or she should indicate the presence or absence of additional sensation or pain. When pain or soreness is found at the first vertebra, the patient is asked to remember this sensation and use it as a guide for pain at other levels.

The examination begins at the 3rd lumbar spinous; after examination of hundreds of patients, this segment appears to be most often neutral. Once the test has begun, the chiropractor stops only to mark the spinous the patient has indicated as painful. Test by placing the thumb *next to* the 3rd lumbar spinous process. It should not be placed *on top of* the spinous. An oscillating motion 3 or 4 times with 4- to 6-pounds of pressure toward the junction of the spinous process and the lamina is to be used. This procedure should continue to all levels listed.

In this manner, the 3rd lumbar, 4th lumbar, 5th lumbar, and reversing, 4th lumbar, 3rd lumbar, 2nd lumbar, 1st lumbar, 12th thoracic, 11th thoracic is tested. The test is completed at the 10th thoracic; after completing one side, the opposite side is tested. Each side is to be marked separately.

(Note: It will be of interest that by far the greatest percentage of spinal level pain is found on the left side.[4])

If the dorsolumbar junction is extremely painful, the physician should not hesitate to examine two or three levels higher. Variations in neural anatomical structures exist and can alter the spinal level of nerve control.[5]

Five possible findings may be present: negative, sensitive, painful, sharp, and highly reactive. One must remember that these are acute and chronic cases, young and old patients, major and minor injuries, single and multiple pain syndromes, and variations in pain tolerance. The chance that all listings are found in one patient is not impossible, but is not likely. If a sensitive and highly reactive level is found on one patient, the highly reactive level would take priority.

The patient declaration of an absence of pain is a negative finding. On rare occasions, a hypersensitive patient will claim that all levels hurt. If this happens, the described technique is performed again, but at a remote level of the spine. Should the same response be noted, the patient is told that the test will be repeated once more. He or she is asked to state the sharpest or most painful area. This usually works quite satisfactorily. **(There will be cases, especially accidents, in which the entire region will be reactive because of the injury. This should not be mistaken for hypersensitivity in the patient. The finding will be in the higher ranges at mostly all levels, in these cases.)**

Segmental Findings

When the spinal segmental level of discomfort or tenderness is listed as sensitive, there are two basic categories.

First, this finding may be present in cases of old underlying, nonreactive pathologies, arthritis, disc degeneration, old fractures, postsurgery, scoliosis, and even certain birth defects.

The second category consists of types A and B.

Type A

- This is the patient with a minor low back injury seen in the office within a few hours or the next day. The injury is not severe enough to cause great soft tissue reactive changes in that short time, hence the segmental findings may show a sensitive rating.

Type B

- This might be the same patient, untreated or treated incorrectly, in whom the condition has persisted for several weeks or months. The original level of injury has progressed through the acute stage and entered a chronic state. Once this occurs, that level is subject to intermittent pain, and during the quiescent period a sensitive finding may be present. Conversely, during the reactive state, a rating of painful, sharp, or highly reactive would be present, and the patient would indicate this verbally.

When painful, joint and associated tissue reaction indicate that either the joint is injured, or associated soft tissue is reactive. This finding is more apt to be found in an older spinal joint lesion that has become slightly reactive, than in a milder injury. It is frequently found associated with those cases having sharp or highly reactive joint and/or soft tissue reaction.

Tissue reaction at the motor unit and paraspinal muscles causing pain indicates that prompt attention is needed. The highly reactive vertebra requires no verbal response from the patient, but it is certain that one will be forthcoming! Flinching or muscle contraction as a protective response will alert the physician to this finding,[6] and ascertains that soft tissue and possibly nerve root inflammation has occurred.

A high reaction at a vertebral level takes precedence over all other recorded reactions acquired during any phase of the examination. The primary treatment will be based upon the spinal level showing the highest reaction to this test. Secondary treatment will be considered, as a followup.

Formulating a differential diagnosis between 5th lumbar motor unit injury and pain from the posterior one third of the lumbosacral junction is often difficult. It is essential, however, to prevent an incorrect diagnosis and treatment that might have little ultimate value to the patient. There are two basic tissues involved that must be considered: the 5th lumbar motor unit including all tissue at the foramen, and the sciatic nerve root, whereas reaction from the posterior one third of this junction may involve ligaments only.

The posterior one third of the lumbosacral junction contains interspinous tissues and, more importantly, the supraspinal ligament that can be extremely painful when injured. The basic difference appears to be related to motion, less than to the extreme range. Although a straight leg raising (SLR) test produces pain to an injured lumbosacral motor unit and nerve root as the pelvis begins to flex, the supraspinal ligament may not be affected until maximum flexion is reached, or flexion under a load that can produce sharp pain at this site. Do not be surprised, however, if the SLR test produces immediate pain to the ligament when the ligament is sufficiently inflamed. Immediate pain might then occur. When injured or under stress, this ligament becomes highly sensitive to pressure, and the 4- to 6-pounds pressure causes immediate pain. When the ligament is normal, that amount of pressure will not produce pain.

In a case in which there is injury to the 5th lumbar motor unit, or nerve, the SLR test produces pain over the lumbosacral junction creating a positive finding. Pain will also be caused at that junction when vertebral testing is conducted. If the supraspinous ligament is not involved, it will be negative to pressure. A negative SLR test and a positive vertebral test indicates old injury or old underlying pathology to the motor unit, without nerve root injury. Injury to the supraspinal ligament may or may not be present. A negative SLR test for the lumbosacral junction indicates no reactive pathology or nerve inflammation at that region. A positive finding may occur when probing the supraspinous ligament. This pain does not involve the motor unit. One must remember that the reaction found at the supraspinal ligament is separate from reaction found at the lumbosacral joint. It should be considered related to the lumbosacral joint only when the SLR test and spinal segmental test at the LS joint and the test to the supraspinal ligament are all positive; even then, with a lumbosacral joint injury present, if highly reactive segments are found from the 3rd lumbar upward to the 10th thoracic, the supraspinal ligament reaction is more apt to be associated with reaction found at the upper spinal segments.

When conducted properly, vertebral testing is a highly accurate method of locating an injured spinal segment regardless of the cause. When this test is coupled with the regional orthopedic low back examination, as described, a formidable foe against low back/leg pain is created. *(All findings must be recorded.)*

Conclusion of the Prone Position

After completing the vertebral tests, a careful manual and visual examination should be done. This type of examination is delayed for two reasons: first, to prevent any pain areas found from influencing the physician's judgment on spinal listings; second, and more importantly, the probing of muscles and tendons could easily change the sensations the patient will be experiencing during vertebral testing. The need for accuracy is critical.

Beginning at the level that has the primary listing, the paraspinal muscles are probed laterally to that level, continuing along the muscle to its lower attachment at the iliac crest. If pain is present at any area along the crest or muscles, it is marked and the location noted. Frequently, this tenderness or pain continues below the crest of the ilium; this area should be marked.

If either of the two posterior pelvic syndromes is present, these areas should also be probed to determine underlying muscle or tendon irritation. As accurate a location as possible must be ascertained for the presence of pain or possible fibrosis. The piriform muscle is often involved at its medial and lateral attachments when the gluteal syndrome is present. The patient with a Thomas syndrome may have pain areas at muscle attachments above and/or posterior to the hip. If the patient has a posterior femoral syndrome or sciatic pain, this is the time to probe for added differentiation. These findings will aid in confirming the previous test. The sciatic notch, and midline down the upper leg is probed; if sciatica is present, pain will be produced—usually very sharp pain. Should the posterior leg pain be diffuse, with no main-line pain on probing, the diagnosis would be posterior femoral syndrome. *(All findings must be recorded.)*

CONCLUSION FOR PHYSICAL EXAMINATION OF LOW BACK/LEG PAIN

The examination for low back/leg pain is concluded. Every effort has been made to test all tissues that might be responsible for low back/leg pain syndromes. **An examination is a tool, a reflection of the physician. It can only reveal what he or she is capable of asking.** There are pain syndromes that can be classified and charted. The knowledge of these syndromes offers a goal or standard, a fixed point that the profession can continue to build upon toward a better diagnostic procedure, and ultimately a more effective treatment.

Segmental Examination Form

The spinal segmental examination form, #111, found in the back of this manual should be used to record the chiropractor's findings. The segmental examination is designed to examine each spinal segment, including the soft tissue capable of showing a reaction to the examination and subject to injury or reaction. These injured or reactive elements cause the symptoms of pain and muscle contraction found in low back/leg pain cases. The various findings found in patients with low back, groin, hip, and leg pain can be recorded on this form for a permanent record. It can also be used when periodic progress reports are necessary.

REFERENCES

1. Peter D: Lumbar nerve root: The enigmatic eponyms. *Spine* 9(1):3, 1984
2. Hadley LA: Intervertebral joint subluxation, bony impingement and foramen encroachment with nerve root changes. *AJR* 26(3):377, 1951
3. Bastron JA, Birkford RG, Brown JR: Tenderness to percussion and deep pressure may supply evidence of radicular irritation. In *Clinical Examination in Neurology,* 2nd ed. Philadelphia, WB Saunders, 1954; p.272
4. Cox JM: *Low Back Pain,* 4th ed. Baltimore, Williams & Wilkins, 1985;p.10
5. Gray H: *Gray's Anatomy,* 30th ed. Philadelphia, Lea & Febiger, 1984;p.1229
6. Mennel JM: *Back Pain,* 1st ed. Boston, Little, Brown & Co, 1960;p.14

Chapter 8

Paraspinal Pain Syndrome

The investigation of a case involving low back pain is both exciting and challenging because it offers many avenues to be explored. There are two primary pain syndromes found in the low back region, the paraspinal and lumbar.[1] These two pain syndromes are occasionally found in the same case, but are most frequently found individually. They may also be associated with other pain syndromes, called composite (multiple) pain syndromes, and when these composites are present they create quite a complicated picture. Each pain syndrome has its individual peculiarities, and for clarification they are best discussed and understood when found alone before any attempt is made to address the more complicated multiples.

PARASPINAL PAIN SYNDROME

Most patients who suffer from a paraspinal pain syndrome are average individuals, for the most part not involved in strenuous activities. A large percentage of these patients are not even aware that their activities created the foundation for low back pain unless the pain immediately follows some action. The term *foundation* is used because many low back cases fall in the category of secondary spinal lesions. A primary spinal lesion produces immediate pain as a result of the forced subluxation/disrelation injury. Secondary spinal lesions are dormant or semidormant lesions that have existed for some period of time, with the body tissues changing slowly. They cause periodic low back problems in varying degrees. These lesions may become acute, reactive, and painful, following added motion, stress, or further injury. The amount of motion or stress does not always appear equivalent to the amount of pain or disability; this is not unusual, particularly for secondary spinal lesions.[2]

As the low back areas of pain are determined, in the precise manner described in the first chapter of this manual,[3] six pain areas are most commonly found within the paraspinal syndrome area, and any one or more may be affected. The chance that pain would entirely encompass the paraspinal pain syndrome area is probably rare, if it ever occurs. Note the general body area of this pain syndrome in Figure 8–1.

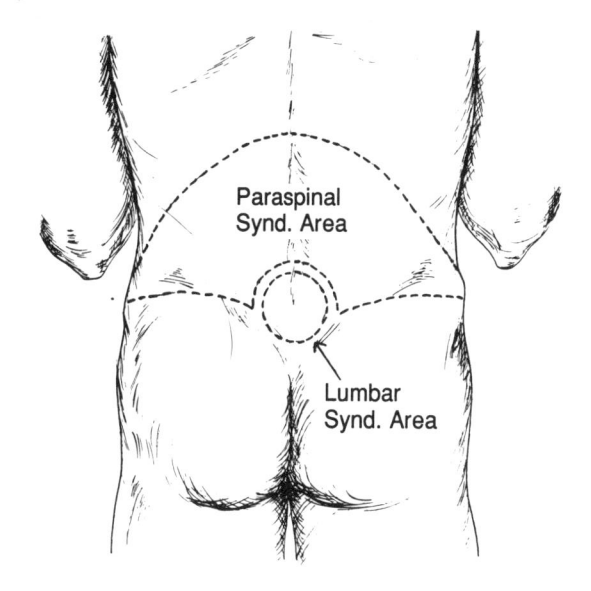

Figure 8–1

Common Areas of Pain Found in This Syndrome

Figures 8–2 through 8–7 show the most common areas of pain found within the boundaries of this syndrome.

1. One area is approximately 2 inches lateral to the 5th lumbar spinous process above the sacroiliac joint. The diameter of this area may range from the size of a quarter to a fifty-cent piece (see Fig. 8–2).
2. Any point along the posterior iliac crests and slightly above or below the crest may have sharp areas of pain, or the pain may extend parallel to the iliac crests in varying lengths (see Fig. 8–3).
3. Pain may be indicated close and parallel to the spine in isolated areas or may extend along the spine in varying lengths (see Fig. 8–4).

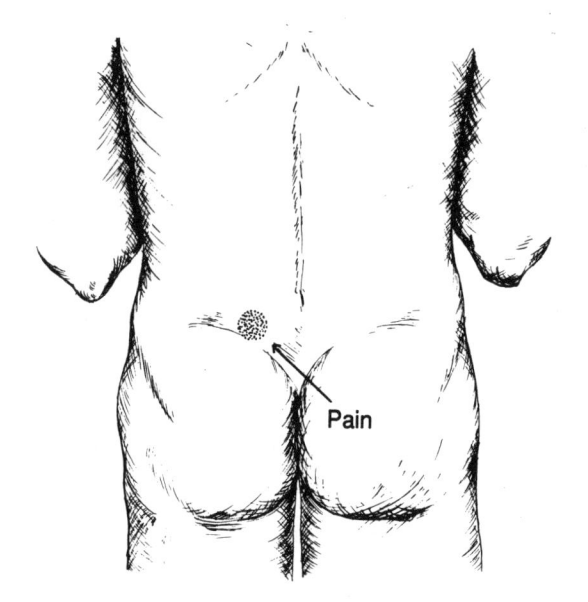

Figure 8–2

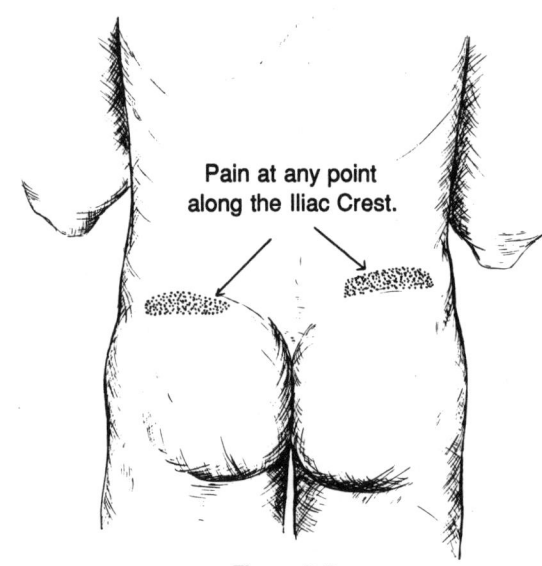

Figure 8–3 Pain at any point along the Iliac Crest.

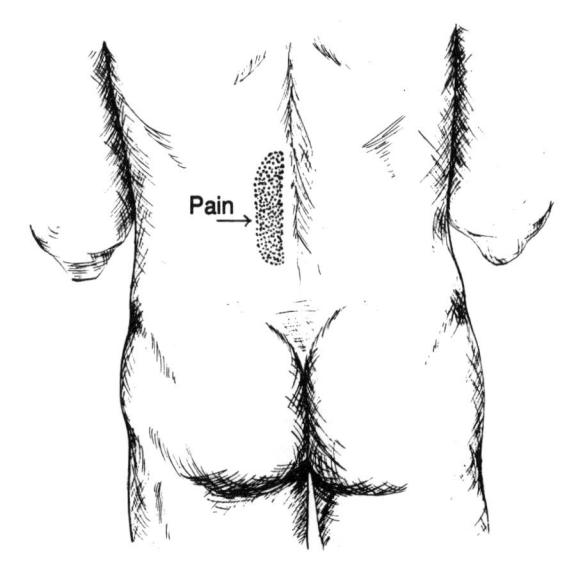

Figure 8–4

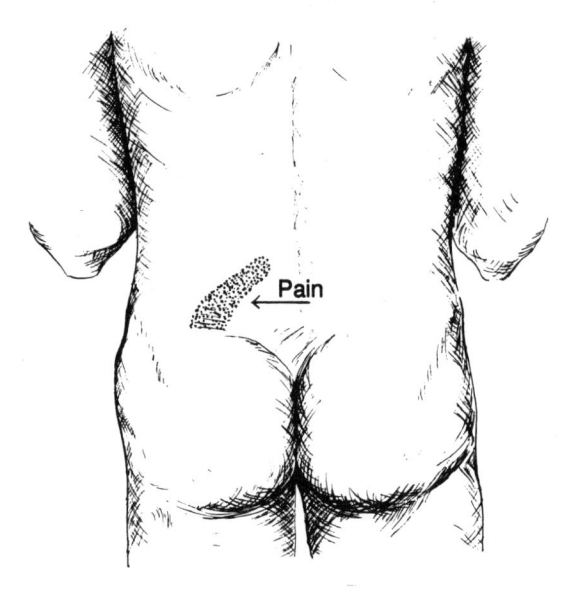

Figure 8–5

4. Two to four inches lateral to the spine pain may be shown similar to no. 3 above (see Fig. 8–5).
5. Pain may be indicated at any low back spinal level (excluding pain over the 5th lumbar and lumbosacral joint) (see Fig. 8–6).
6. An area of pain may be found at the extreme lateral posterior border of the iliac crest (see Fig. 8–7).

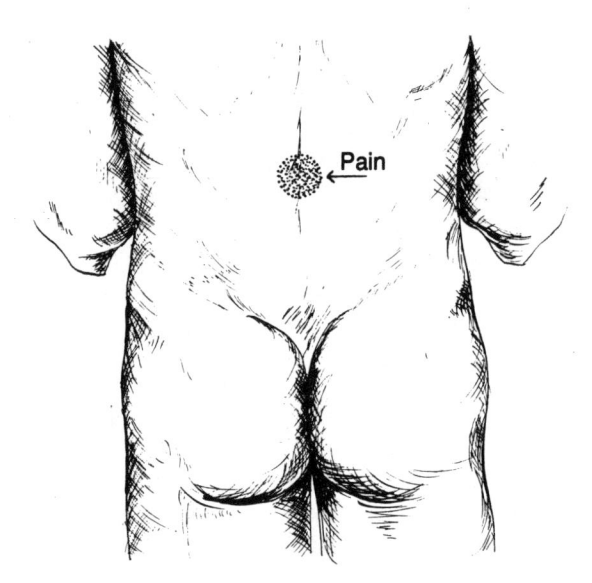

Figure 8–6

One, or more, or even all these pain areas may be present in any given case; they still constitute the **paraspinal pain syndrome.** An understanding of the spinal protective mechanism as described in Chapter 5 permits the chiropractor to visualize why these different locations of pain might be present.

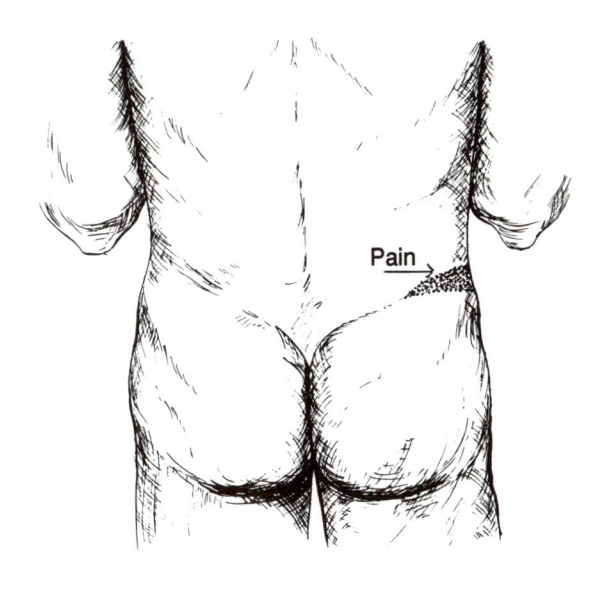

Figure 8–7

Physicians are all aware that patients suffer from low back pain, that pain is a subjective symptom, a symptom that cannot be felt, seen, or recorded with instrumentation. Yet, hundreds of patients from all walks of life can describe the same pain areas. When pain areas are recorded within the perimeters of a pain syndrome, they are classified as that pain syndrome. With their areas of pain recorded on a graph, the perimeters of these pain syndromes then create the permanent visual record.

When it has been determined that the pain areas are truly a paraspinal pain syndrome, the characteristics of this syndrome are then apparent.

Nerve Supply to This Syndrome Area

When becoming reactive to spinal joint injury, the posterior divisions of the spinal nerves, the posterior primary rami, cause antalgic contraction of those muscles supplied, for the purpose of spinal protection.[4] The skin, muscles, and their attachments can become painful as a result. Certain exceptions as discussed in previous chapters include smaller portions of the anterior primary rami nerves. The principle spinal levels of these nerves range from the 10th thoracic to the 2nd lumbar.

Characteristics

The reactive paraspinal pain syndrome is found predominantly in the male, 63%, and 37% in the female. It appears that 66% of the cases are acute and 34% are chronic.

The types of injuries are found in the following percentages:

1. Unknown   34%
2. Twisting   29%
3. Lifting   27%
4. Bending   11%
5. Falls   6%
6. Struck   4%
7. Push–pull   2%

The spinal levels of injury or reaction found by the spinal segmental examination are

1. 12th thoracic   69%
2. 5th lumbar   8%
3. 4th lumbar   1%
4. 12T & 5L   14%
5. 12T & 4L   4%
6. Other levels   8%

The total number injured or reactive for each spinal level are

1. 12th thoracic   86%
2. 5th lumbar   22%
3. 4th lumbar   5%

The previous figures were taken from cases in a retirement community where the average age is 56 years. These figures would probably vary to some degree if determined within an industrial, farming, mining, or college community.

Following the identification of the paraspinal pain syndrome, it is appropriate to conduct both the orthopedic regional examination and the spinal segmental examination, both of which are required to increase knowledge of the case presented, and to determine the spinal segmental level causing the pain syndrome. The injured or reactive spinal levels can be determined by the specific spinal segmental examination, when conducted as shown in Chapter 7. The relationship between the pain syndrome and spinal levels recorded as injured or reactive is so precise that the individual nerve or nerve groups can usually be projected.

Those cases in which the pain area is closely confined to the spinal joint level, as shown in Figure 8–6, rarely create a problem in the determination of the injured spinal level. Even in the pain area shown in Figure 8–4, it should not be too difficult to locate the general lesion level. The spinal segmental examination isolates the actual injured or reactive spinal joint level. When the pain area is away from the spine as shown in Figures 8–2, 8–3, 8–5, and 8–7, and no area of pain is over the reactive segment or close to it, the determination of the precise level of joint injury or reaction becomes more complicated. These areas of pain indicate involvement of muscles that attach to the spine at one end and to the pelvis at the other. Pain may be found in the skin and body of the muscle or only in its attachments along the iliac crest. In more severe cases, the pain areas may run together along the iliac crest, or from the iliac crest to the spine, and would not then be recognized as separate areas.

The patient observed whose body trunk is flexed to one side has a contraction of the quadratus lumborum muscle with the neural activity at the spine sufficient to cause these muscles to react. Pain may be found at multiple areas.

The primary nerve levels most responsible for the paraspinal pain syndrome end at the 1st lumbar nerve.[5] Review of the reactive spinal levels show that the thoracolumbar is the primary level injured or reactive. This leaves about 25% injured or reactive findings at the 4th and 5th lumbar. These levels relate to the paraspinal pain syndrome via the body's protective mechanism, causing stimulation or reaction to the posterior primary rami activating those muscles to limit motion, for joint protection.

Chapter 5, Pain Mechanism, discusses the connection.[6] This information is a hypothesis of how injury, disease, birth defects, etc., of lower lumbar spinal segments may send neural impulses in varying degrees to those nerve fibers capable of causing muscle antalgic contraction for protective splinting. It appears that if these neural impulses reach a certain level or are continuous, they become an adverse influence to those spinal levels receiving them and may even be responsible for a pathological entity at those levels.[7] Paraspinal pain results from this continuous bombardment of nerve impulses and the impulses may be transferred to the anterior primary nerve division.[8] If this occurs, pain syndromes can appear in areas remote from the spine. This is not inconceivable. Referred pain such as angina due to coronary spasm is common, as are many other referred pain areas. In low back cases, the difference is that the nerve endings responsible for pain at specific areas are caused by irritation or injury to the spinal nerve root, thus making a direct connection, and the resulting action is related to a normal body function—*protection*.[9] This must be kept in mind as the patient is examined to clarify the reason(s) certain spinal levels may react in unexpected ways.

EXAMINATION FINDING FOR THE PARASPINAL PAIN SYNDROME

The single test that has been misused, or its erratic findings misunderstood, is the SLR test.

This test is highly effective in the determination of the paraspinal pain syndrome when combined with the spinal segmental examination.

A negative SLR test tells us that the lumbosacral joint is not reactive and that although pain is present in the paraspinal region, its muscle involvement does not extend to those muscles and attachments connected to the pelvis. The muscles probably involved in this type case are those associated with only the spinal segments.

A positive SLR test must be considered in two ways.

1. Positive at the lumbosacral joint. This indicates lumbosacral joint injury or reaction. This is not a common finding when only paraspinal pain syndromes are present.
2. Positive finding—pain in those muscles and/or their attachments that arise from the spine and attach to the iliac crest. This finding is common when paraspinal pain syndrome areas are present and indicate that the spinal protective mechanism is activated by antalgic contraction.

When pain exists outside the boundaries of the 5th lumbar and lumbosacral joint, the findings are commonly listed as a positive SLR test, but generally considered for lesions of the 5th lumbar or lumbosacral joint. If indicated for those joints, the interpretation is incorrect.

The SLR test is limited. It tells us that muscles and/or tendons of motion are reactive or hypersensitive. Pain may be present before these tissues begin to react in a degree sufficient to respond for simple testing procedures. In that event, the SLR test could be negative and might leave the impression that the pain suffered by the patient is either unimportant, or minor at best. The SLR test does not always indicate the integrity of the spinal motor unit, particularly those segments above the 4th lumbar vertebra. It is true that it may aid in the determination of 5th lumbar lesions, but the spinal segmental examination is necessary to confirm or reject this finding. The spinal segmental examination is the definitive test capable of proving or disproving the existence of an active or reactive spinal joint lesion and its level of activity.

Examples

The following is a hypothetical case in which the patient has a paraspinal lesion. The woman has pain at an area slightly above the right iliac crest, about 3 to 4 inches lateral to the 5th lumbar spine. The pain is sharp, principally on movement. It prevents the patient from carrying out her duties as a clerk in a drive-in grocery where speed is necessary to fill orders and she must gather the groceries from shelves placed on various levels. The pain's onset was 8 days earlier and had finally progressed to the point that she was forced to see a chiropractor. Her age is 35 years, she is 5 feet 2 inches tall, weighing 127 lbs. When asked if she has had previous low back problems, she stated that she had been in an auto accident 10 years previously and suffered minor low back problems for a short period of time (untreated). She experienced no problems since then until she began working at this job. At this point, it is best not to prognosticate the diagnosis or become biased toward a certain direction until the entire regional orthopedic examination has been completed.

The SLR test is then initiated. No pain is caused by raising the patient's right leg; *Negative R* is recorded. When the left leg is raised to about 70°, the patient indicates that pain is caused on the right side, at the same spot as she originally experienced it. *Positive L 70—over right iliac crest* is recorded. No other area of pain is produced by this test.

It has been learned from this test that there is no active 5th lumbar lesion—no center line pain caused by the SLR test. Additionally, the direction of pelvic tilt rather than the leg appears to be responsible for the increased pain at the right iliac crest. Either the right or left leg might have produced a positive finding. With these findings, followed by a positive spinal segmental test only at the 12th thoracic—1st lumbar segment, it could be assumed that the patient suffers from an uncomplicated paraspinal pain syndrome. This would be true even if an x-ray showed some degeneration at another spinal level, with a negative finding for the spinal segmental examination. (Gross spinal pathology should not be accepted as a cause of pain until that segmental level is proven reactive to examination.)

Other test findings can also be considered for the same case.

- The right leg is raised, some pain is noted at the lumbosacral joint; *Pos. R 75°—LS Joint. Slight* is recorded.
- The left leg is raised, with slight pain to the LS joint. *Pos. L 80—LS Joint. Slight* is recorded.
- No increase in the right iliac pain area. *Pain area test neg.* is recorded.

These findings provide an entirely different evaluation in the presence of the same pain syndrome.

The first clue to low back pain complications in this case is the positive SLR test at the pain-free lumbosacral joint. The implications are that a 5th lumbar low-reactive secondary lesion is present. Even this should not be prejudged because the pain may arise from the supraspinal ligament as a result of thoracolumbar torsion. The spinal segmental examination offers another indicator for the evaluation of this problem, and of course lumbar x-rays assist. This case is, obviously, no longer an uncomplicated paraspinal pain syndrome.

There may also be the following findings.

- The right leg is raised with no back pain. *Neg. R* is recorded.
- The left leg is raised with no back pain. *Neg. L* is recorded.

The spinal segment examination produces a sensitive reaction at both the 5th lumbar and 12th thoracic levels. This is a case that falls somewhere between the previous cases. A low-grade secondary lesion is probably at the 5th lumbar level, sending signals to the lumbar plexus. The 12th thoracic segment could be a low-grade primary lesion. This configuration would be more accurate because a paraspinal rather than the lumbar syndrome is present. A case of this type requires treatment at both levels, but it is necessary to ensure that primary treatment is at the 12th thoracic level due to the presence of the paraspinal pain syndrome.

The actual time required for testing this patient does not exceed 10 minutes. The information acquired from the tests, when conducted with care, in their proper sequence, and associated with the understanding of the findings, is well-worth the time spent.

Discussion Related to Treatment

Of the eight major pain syndromes, this syndrome area is the only one where pain can be shown to exist in a variety of locations within it. Moreover, the primary lesion levels for this condition range from the 10th thoracic to the 1st lumbar, but less frequent spinal levels of injury causing this pain syndrome may exist as high as the 8th thoracic and as low as the 3rd lumbar.

Because of the many levels that can be involved and the fact that either a primary or one or more secondary lesions may exist, and that this spinal range of segments includes vertebral joints that differ in their ability to function within normal ranges of motion, the physician is confronted with a potential problem that seems almost impossible to resolve.

In those cases in which one or two of these joints are reactive to the examination, those joints should be treated by specific spinal segmental adjustments and manipulation, ordinarily preceded by some form of treatment such as diathermy, or ultrasound, depending upon the type of lesion. The tissue must be relaxed as much as is possible.

Paraspinal pain syndromes are caused not only by joint injury, but by muscle response related to the spinal protective mechanism. This muscle reaction may be only a small group of muscles associated with two or three spinal segments. It may also involve, however, longer spinal muscles extending to several segments, and other groups of muscles related to regional motion. The physician should recognize that if an attempt is made to treat all the muscles or groups of muscles as individual injuries, progress would ensue very slowly, if at all. The examination, particularly the segmental examination, will locate the most reactive joints. These are the joints to be treated and the treatment must start at the highest reactive joints, continuing to lesser reactive joints as each joint reaction subsides.

This condition can be found associated with any other pain syndrome, and when other syndromes are present it should nevertheless be considered a priority condition for treatment because it indicates that the protective spinal mechanism is reactive. Other pain syndromes that are present may also be a result of the antalgic muscle contraction. Once this condition is reduced and controlled, other pain syndromes can then be addressed, should they continue to exist.

In conclusion, the author believes the importance of precise classification and examination procedures in all low back/leg pain cases from spinal lesions and the recording of those records is necessary for a proper pretreatment diagnostic work-up, and essential for any third parties that might become involved.

REFERENCES

1. Thomas JE: Classification of low back/leg pain syndromes, Part 2. *FCA Journal* November–December: p.18, 1985
2. Thomas JE: Classification of low back/leg pain syndromes, Part 4. *FCA Journal* March–April:p.32,1986
3. Thomas JE: Classification of low back/leg pain syndromes, Part 2. *FCA Journal* November–December: p.18, 1985
4. Wood J: Acute locked facet syndrome and its treatment by manipulation under local periarticular anesthesia—Part 1: Clinical perspective and pilot study proposal. *JMPT* 7(4):211, 1984
5. Gray H: *Gray's Anatomy,* 30th ed. Philadelphia, Lea & Febiger, 1984;p.466
6. Thomas JE: Classification of low back/leg pain syndromes, Part 5. *FCA Journal* July–August:p.32,1986
7. Rydevik B, Brown M, Lundborg G: Pathoanatomy and pathophysiology of nerve root compression. *Spine* 9(1): 7, 1984
8. Wood L: Acute locked facet syndrome and its treatment by manipulation under local periarticular anesthesia—Part 1: Clinical perspective and pilot study proposal. *JMPT* 7(4):211, 1984
9. Pressman AH, Nickles SL: Neurophysiological and nutritional consideration of pain control. *JMPT* 7(4): 219, 1984

Chapter 9

Lumbar Pain Syndrome

For the past three or four decades, lesions found at the 4th or 5th lumbar spinal level have been considered responsible for almost all low back/leg pain caused by spinal lesions. By those physicians who maintain this concept, the primary lesion considered for this devastation is thought to result from injury to or destruction of the spinal disc at the 5th lumbar. Generally, it is thought that 90% of lumbar pains are related to changes of function of the 4th and 5th lumbar discs and these various changes of the discs result in low back or leg pain.[1] Although authors of such information may well know that there are many cases that do not fall within this category, the reader, particularly young doctors looking for causes, may take this type of statement at face value. Adhering to this concept has been very difficult, as the true areas of pain suffered by the patient do not conform to dermatome patterns and pertain to almost half the body area. The ability of many patients to move in varied directions is not compatible with true disc lesions and this causes some concern. The fact is that present physical and x-ray (CAT scan, MRI) examination procedures do not result in consistent findings, thus creating frustration for many chiropractors treating low back/leg pain cases. The final irony is that the treating chiropractor has many patients who do not fit the definition(s) regardless of multidirectional descriptions of disc lesions. This complex pain syndrome is discussed below.

LUMBAR PAIN SYNDROME

The lumbar syndrome is a small pain area over the 5th lumbar spinal segment and lumbosacral joint. In some cases, it may extend slightly below the lumbosacral joint. This area is the smallest pain syndrome of all, but certainly not the least in its effect on the patient. In most cases, the area is approximately 2 to 2½ inches in diameter (see Fig. 9–1).[1–4]

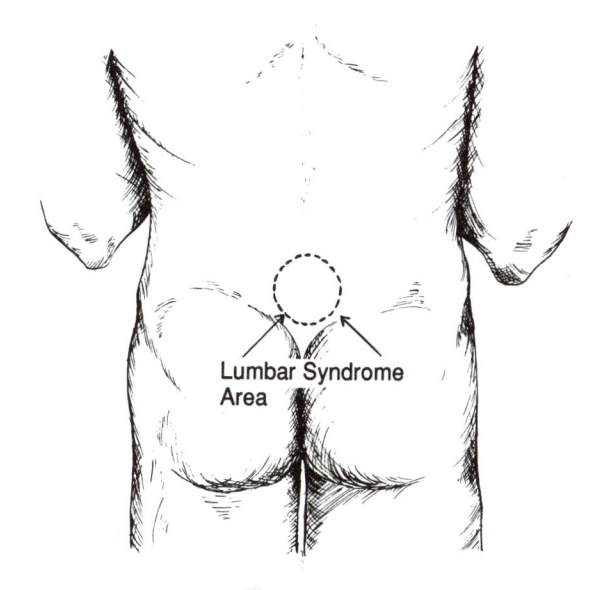

Figure 9–1

Spinal lesions at this level are responsible for reactions at either or both the anterior and posterior primary neural rami.[5,6] The presence of the lumbar pain syndrome indicates injury or reaction to only the posterior primary rami from that level. Pain to the posterior femoral pain syndrome area or down the back of the leg shows that the anterior primary rami is activated. In that case, however, it would not be considered a single lumbar pain syndrome.

Like other secondary spinal lesions, disc pathology may be associated with the lumbar syndrome. As previously mentioned, a disc lesion is a secondary spinal lesion, capable under certain circumstances of causing pain via joint changes. The disc, per se, cannot cause pain, but when it degenerates or loses mass it changes the relationship of the facets. Ordinarily, this change is quite slow, allowing the body to accept the facet changes without a protective body reaction. Slow, abnormal changes in the disc can and do result in periodic low-grade back pain from facet jamming, which causes lumbar pain syndromes. The diagnosis is facet jamming.

The most important objective in the evaluation of the lumbar pain syndrome is the differential diagnosis between the 5th lumbar facet injury, reaction, or both, and the supraspinal ligament injury, reaction, or both. Careful segmental examination of the 5th lumbar and the ligament indicates which tissue is reactive.

Lesions at this level are responsible for the antalgic protective muscular response found in the low back region, arising from higher spinal levels.[7,8] Pain syndromes from the lumbar plexus, anterior primary, or posterior primary rami, may also be a result from 5th lumbar lesions via nerve impulses shunting from one rami to the other.[9] This is frequently seen in cases in which the posterior femoral nerve is irritated and painful. This is discussed in the section on the posterior femoral pain syndrome.

Area of Pain Found in This Syndrome

1. An area of pain approximately 2 to 2½ inches in diameter over the 5th lumbar spinal segment and lumbosacral joint.
2. A second area may be superimposed over the area described above and may occasionally extend slightly below the lumbosacral joint. The primary difference between this and the previous pain area is not location, but the tissues involved. During the spinal segmental examination, these two pain areas must be differentiated, as the diagnosis and treatment may differ for each area.

(Whether or not these pain areas can be separated at the time they are located, they nevertheless constitute the *lumbar syndrome*.)

Nerve Supply to This Syndrome Area

The nerve supply to this syndrome is much like the nerve supply to the paraspinal syndrome in that it represents reaction from the posterior primary rami nerves arising from lower lumbar segments and may extend into sacral segments in the more severe cases of deep muscle contraction. When reactive, 12th thoracic/1st lumbar nerves may cause cutaneous pain over that area. The primary local response from the muscles is protective, reducing motion to the lumbosacral joint.

Characteristics

The lumbar syndrome has been found to exist in 28% of all single-pain cases. Industrial, farm, mining, and college communities may show slightly different ranges.

This syndrome affects 68% of males and 32% of female.[9] It is acute in 78% of all cases and chronic in 22%.

The types of known injuries are as follows.

1. Lifting 30%
2. Unknown 28%
3. Twisting 21%
4. Bending 12%
5. Falls 8%
6. Push–pull 4%
7. Struck 2%

It is interesting to note that lifting does not, as popularly thought, constitute a larger share than the total of other causes. Twisting and bending accidents are common. Heavy weights in excess of 40 pounds do not appear often enough to be of specific importance. The unknown cases appear close to the 30% range, similar to those figures found in the paraspinal syndrome.

Spinal levels injured or reactive found by the segmental spinal examination are

1. 12th thoracic 21%
2. 5th lumbar 54%
3. 4th lumbar 10%
4. 5th and 12T 16%
5. 4th and 12T 3%
6. other 8%

Total number injured or reactive for each spinal level are listed below.

1. 5th lumbar 70%
2. 12th thoracic 39%
3. 4th lumbar 13%

In the paraspinal pain syndrome, about 25% of the injured or reactive spinal segments are found at the 5th lumbar level. In the lumbar pain syndrome, the examination of spinal segments indicates that almost half the spinal levels involved in these cases are found at the 12th thoracic. This would tend to reenforce the hypothesis that nerve impulses from the lower lumbar area activate the spinal nerves supplying low back muscles that are capable of producing antalgic contraction for spinal protection, and may show an association with the second, superimposed pain area. There is an unusual situation in this syndrome, in that a second pain area may overlay that caused by injury or reaction to the 5th lumbar or lumbosacral joint. This second pain area appears to arise from the supraspinal ligament, and may be present without injury or reaction from the 5th lumbar spinal segment. (Note Fig. 9–2.) The pressure points for a differential diagnosis are close: but careful digital examination with 4 to 6 pounds pressure will show the separation of reaction. If both are reactive, it indicates both 5th

Supraspinous Ligt.
5L Spinous Process
Pressure Points 1-2

1. For 5L Lesion
2. For Supraspinous Ligt. React.

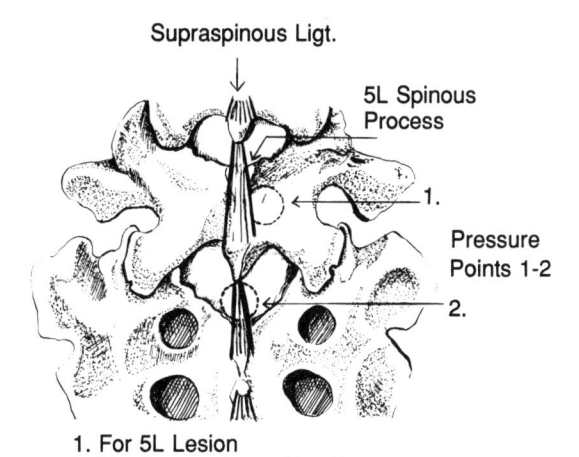

Figure 9–2

lumbar joint injury and supraspinal ligament injury or reaction.

When this second pain area is present, it is indistinguishable from the first pain area by either the patient or doctor and requires a combination of findings from the orthopedic and spinal segmental examination to formulate the differential diagnosis. If this determination is not made, inaccurate findings occur and unnecessary or ineffective treatment is highly probable, with increased costs and possible disability.

This superimposed pain area had been undetected until the spinal segmental examination was combined with the precise regional orthopedic examination. Awareness of this pain overlay has answered some questions about the lumbar syndrome, but poses others. It enables us to understand the reason a positive SLR test can be present without the existence of a true 5th lumbar lesion. It also gives us a better insight into the ability of the patient to be active in almost all movements regardless of an apparent lumbosacral lesion, and why repeated movement can fatigue the low back supporting tissue, causing a delayed increase in pain, again without a true 4th or 5th lumbar motor unit lesion. Questions do arise as to the cause of pain at the supraspinal ligament, particularly when the 4th, or 5th, or both lumbar segments are nonreactive.

It might be understandable if the primary cause of this lumbar syndrome were the lifting of heavy weights, thus causing an axial injury to the lumbosacral joint, or if the patient had been working in a flexed position for periods of time. This is not the case. The pain area is not always present with a 5th lumbar lesion, but it is frequently present without indications of a lumbosacral active lesion. Clinical study for this area has shown that specific spinal manipulation at the thoracolumbar spinal level has been most effective in reducing the lumbar syndrome pain in many cases, and particularly so when little or no segmental reaction is found at the lumbosacral joint.[3] Pain caused by injury or reaction to the 5th lumbar spinal level is found over that segment and the lumbosacral joint when neural stimulation does not activate other pain syndromes. When the patient indicates, by following the physician's guidelines, that a lumbar pain syndrome is present, the next step is to conduct the regional examination.

Examination Findings for the Lumbar Pain Syndrome

One test in this examination, the straight leg raising (SLR) test, is of prime importance for the determination of 5th lumbar active or reactive lesions. When the SLR test is negative, no pain produced, or no increase in pain noted, a nonreactive status at the 5th lumbar motor unit is indicated, regardless of x-ray evidence showing gross pathology to this joint.

Birth defects, arthritis, previous lesions, and so on, can be present at the lumbosacral joint, may be visible in the x-ray field, and remain in a nonactive status. Being nonactive does not prevent this pathological entity from sending low-grade neural signals to nerves supplying muscles capable of producing antalgic contraction. When positive spinal segmental findings at the 5th lumbar are associated with the negative SLR test, we can be reasonably assured that neurologic signals are being sent out. Antalgic contraction may be present at the 4th and 5th lumbar segments involving the deep muscles, not causing a positive SLR test, but able to produce increased pain and contraction when activated by increased body motion. This configuration seems to be present in many patients who are relatively pain free with remissions of pain when active (less than normal).

It becomes increasingly evident that the physician must be aware of the difference between active and reactive joints and the part they play in the pain syndromes suffered by the patient. With the proper examination procedures, this knowledge also gives an indication as to the spinal level that requires treatment.

The SLR test is positive *only* when pain at the 5th lumbar or lumbosacral joint is increased. **Pain over any other area should not be considered as a positive SLR test for this syndrome.** Other areas of pain caused by the SLR test could be, for the most part, associated with latent paraspinal or other pain syndromes, and should of course be investigated. A positive or negative SLR test may be found in either or both lumbar pain syndromes, but the meaning is different.

The spinal segmental examination must be used to differentiate the two pain syndromes. When there is both a positive SLR test and positive spinal segmental findings at the 5th lumbar joint, then one must consider the 5th lumbar an active lesion. A negative for both tests would eliminate an active lumbar lesion and indicate the presence of the second pain area. A negative finding over the supraspinal ligament during the spinal segmental examination eliminates that pain syndrome. Because variations do occur, experience is important, and as stated before, the most acute spinal segmental finding should take precedence. An active 5th lumbar lesion requires x-rays to help classify the lesion as primary or secondary. The type of manipulation and associated treatment can then be considered.

A positive SLR test (at the 5th lumbar) with negative spinal segmental findings is rare, but may be found within a few hours following the injury. This ordinarily occurs before the soft tissue becomes reactive, or may result from delays in soft tissue reaction due to a chronic status. When the injury is superimposed upon constitutional disease of bone, previous injury, or defect, existing damage to the soft tissue may delay or prevent a normal response. In some cases, the injury is not severe enough for segmental reaction. Tissues that are in a chronic state from previous injury, or suffer changes from constitutional disease of bone, tend to be erratic in their ability to respond in a normal fashion.

Because, in single pain syndromes, injury to the 5th lumbar spinal level only accounts for approximately 6% of anterior primary rami reaction (posterior femoral/sciatic syndromes), and yet its overall presence is second for all low back/leg pain syndromes, the chiropractor must realize that posterior primary neural injury and/or reaction is of major importance.

When the lumbar syndrome is the only pain syndrome present, all the spinal reaction is in a localized area. The level of reaction for the SLR and spinal segmental tests should be a guide to the severity of the lesion in most cases. The physician must then evaluate the history and x-ray findings to determine whether the lesion is primary or secondary. When the spinal segmental examination is conducted and the 12th thoracic segment is hypersensitive, the suspicion that neural impulses may be coming from the 5th lumbar lesion is raised. This consideration should then be added to the information regarding the lesion.

This information should appear as noted below.

1. Lumbar syndrome, no other pain area
2. Primary or secondary lesion
3. Reaction rating for SLR test at 5L motor unit
4. Reaction rating for spinal segmental test at 5th L
5. Reaction rating for spinal segmental test at 12th T
6. Reaction rating for other spinal segments

Examples

1. Lumbar syndrome (solo)
2. Primary lesion
3. SLR—increased pain—not sharp (5th L motor unit)
4. Seg—exam—5th L—sensitive
5. Seg—exam—12th T—neg
6. Seg—exam—other seg neg

This information would indicate that the patient suffers from a localized 5th lumbar lesion, not reactive enough to send signals to the nerves for antalgic protection, and that local muscle contraction and reaction from soft tissue are at a minimum.

Another case may read in this way.

1. Lumbar syndrome (solo)
2. Secondary lesion
3. SLR—increased pain—sharp—30° (5th L motor unit)
4. Seg—exam—5th L—highly reactive
5. Seg—exam—12th T—sharp pain
6. Seg—exam—other seg 1st L sensitive

This is the same pain syndrome with different findings and classification of the lesion. Obviously one does not expect to control or correct these cases with the same treatments. There is certainly nothing mysterious about these differences once the chiropractor is able to ascertain what makes the difference. It also accounts for the possibility that one case requires a minimum of treatments, whereas another requires a maximum number although the syndromes on the surface are identical. These are the differences that the physician and third party payors would like to know, or should know, and which need to be known when total bills for patients vary a great deal with the same pain syndrome or spinal subluxation lesion. These differences are not unusual for spinal pathology or injury any more than are all cardiac lesions the same or every case of diabetes is identical.

Below is one more example.

1. Lumbar syndrome (solo)
2. No motor unit lesion detected
3. SLR—neg (5th L motor unit)

4. Seg—exam—5th L—over supraspinous ligament—sharp pain
5. Seg—exam—12th T—neg
6. Seg—exam—other segments—neg

This case is also a lumbar pain syndrome, but involves different tissues. The 5th lumbar motor unit appears intact and normal, with the reactive tissue found only at the supraspinal ligament. In most cases, treatment is not required at the 5th lumbar segment.

Differential Diagnosis from the Sacroiliac Lesion

There must be a differentiation made in some cases between the lumbar syndrome and lesions from injury to the sacroiliac joint, because occasionally the two have similar pain symptoms. In most cases of a lumbar syndrome, the pain does not extend over the sacrum, but there are exceptions. In most cases of chronic sacroiliac lesions, the pain does not extend into the lumbar syndrome space, but again, there are exceptions. The basic examination will generally detect the difference.

Sacroiliac joint lesions generally fall into two types.

Type A

- This type of sacroiliac lesion is usually caused by lifting or a fall, with immediate pain. It is frequently so devastating that the patient is not ambulatory. Severe pain is found over most of the posterior pelvic area and often into the hip and leg. When they present, these patients are usually using crutches or have other people to help them. Pressure to the sacroiliac joint causes extreme pain.

Type B

- The second type most apt to be found in the chiropractor's office is the chronic case and/or those cases where slippage at this joint is relatively minor; although it may be extremely painful, the patient is ambulatory. Severe leg pain is not usually associated with these cases, but when it is present it generally relates to portions of the posterior femoral pain syndrome area. This is not unexpected, because the cluneal nerve, particularly the inferior cluneal fibers at that area, is closely associated with the sacroiliac joint as are the posterior femoral nerve and sciatic nerve. Careful probing of the sacroiliac joint produces additional pain to the entire length of that joint. Along the joint, this sharp pain is not present in a lumbar pain syndrome.

In chronic and lesser injured cases, the pain surrounds the sacroiliac joint involving the posterior primary rami nerves at the 5th lumbar and sacral level. It may in some cases be close to and/or include the muscle attachments at the iliac crest near the joint, and activates the protective mechanism related to the deep paraspinal muscles. Antalgic contraction of both lower lumbar attachments and those muscular attachments to the sacrum and even the hip may be involved. The best views of these attachments are probably found in *Manual Medicine*.[11]

It is important to be aware that, because the sacroiliac joint is large, injuries causing a subluxation to this joint may well cause a subluxation lesion at the lumbosacral joint and even joints above this level. Changes to the kinesiology due to injuries of this joint could also affect other joints and may be much slower in developing.

Four to six pounds of digital pressure against the joint, producing sharp pain at it, is the best indication for the diagnosis of this lesion. The physician places his or her thumb on the sacrum, pushing laterally against the lip of the ilium, beginning at the bottom and working upward. If a joint lesion is present it will cause pain. The opposite joint is examined for comparison, keeping in mind that a sacroiliac slip on one side may affect the opposite joint, but not as much.

Lifting the leg with the patient in the prone position and simultaneously pressing downward on the sacroiliac joint may also give some indication of a joint lesion due to increased pain at the joint. Lowering the leg off the table with the patient in a supine position may increase the joint pain (Gaenslen's Test). The pressure technique at the joint appears to be the most accurate; with confirmation from the other tests, a sacroiliac lesion can be diagnosed, but the basic orthopedic and spinal segmental tests should not be omitted.

DISCUSSION RELATED TO TREATMENT

In thinking about treatment for the lumbar pain syndrome, the two basic causes for this pain must be considered.

1. A lesion only to the lumbosacral joint
2. A lesion above this joint causing the supraspinous ligament to react

(Both factors may be in evidence.)

Also, the chiropractor should consider the status of the joint in those cases where it is the causative factor. Primary lesions to this joint when it is not causing radicular pain, as is found in this syndrome, are usually less difficult to correct than are secondary lesions, depending upon the severity of the case. The physician must remember that this lesion in this type of case, primary, or secondary, is not great enough to produce reaction to the anterior primary rami, thus permitting a good prognosis in most instances.

According to the database for hundreds of cases, reaction from the 4th lumbar, using 4 to 6 pounds of pressure, is only present in 13% of those cases; thus, when the 5th lumbar is the only reactive joint, it is the only joint that requires treatment with specific segmental manipulation. When the 12th thoracic–1st lumbar are involved, both areas must be treated, but the 12th thoracic–1st lumbar must first be treated as the primary lesion. Obviously, it is necessary to first reduce any factor that might play a part in 5th lumbar joint disrelation. The reduction of the supraspinous ligament pain with continued pain to the joint then demands attention to that joint. Reduced pain to the 12th thoracic–1st lumbar is the first clue that treatment should be successful.

The evaluation or diagnosis of low back leg/pain is not simply the knowledge that the patient has pain somewhere in that general area, nor that the cause or reaction is always the same or similar. It requires the ability of the chiropractor to segregate each pain syndrome and carefully investigate all its ramifications. Those doctors treating low back/leg pain syndromes should be as precise in their procedures as possible.

REFERENCES

1. Thomas JE: Classification of low back/leg pain syndromes, Part 2. *FCA Journal* November–December: p.18, 1985
2. Thomas JE: Classification of low back/leg pain syndromes, Part 3. *FCA Journal* January–February: p.37, 1986
3. Thomas JE: Classification of low back/leg pain syndromes, Part 4. *FCA Journal* March-April:p.32, 1986
4. Thomas JE: Classification of low back/leg pain syndromes—pain syndromes, Part 4 of a series (Part 2). *FCA Journal* May–June:p.38, 1986
5. Hamilton WJ: *Textbook of Human Anatomy,* 2nd ed. St. Louis MO, CV Mosby Co, 1976;p.138
6. Rydevik B, Brown M, Lundborg G: Pathoanatomy and pathophysiology of nerve root compression. *Spine* 9(1):7, 1984
7. Pressman AH, Nickles SL: Neurophysiological and nutritional consideration of pain control. *JMPT* 7(4):219, 1984
8. Thomas JE: Classification of low back/leg pain syndromes, Part 5. *FCA Journal* July–August:p.32, 1986
9. Wood L: Acute locked facet syndrome and its treatment by manipulation under local periarticular anesthesia—Part 1: Clinical perspective and pilot study proposal. *JMPT* 7(4):211, 1984
10. Thomas JE: Classification of low back/leg pain syndromes—Pain syndromes, Part 4 of a series (Part 2). *FCA Journal* May–June:p.38, 1986
11. Dvorak J, Dvorak V: General overview and list of the different muscles. *Manual Medicine.* Stuttgart-New York, Thieme-Stratton Inc. 1984;p.156

Chapter 10

Inguinal Pain Syndrome

The inguinal pain syndrome is not a low back pain problem; it is, however, a nerve syndrome arising from irritation or injury to spinal nerves, therefore, properly designated a member of the low back/leg pain spinal syndromes.[1]

INGUINAL PAIN SYNDROME

This pain syndrome is an area found in the pelvic region and is most frequently caused by a subluxation/disrelation lesion at a spinal motor unit. Note the three regions found in Chapter 1, Figure 1–1. This area extends around the body to include the anterior body area as shown in Figure 10–1.

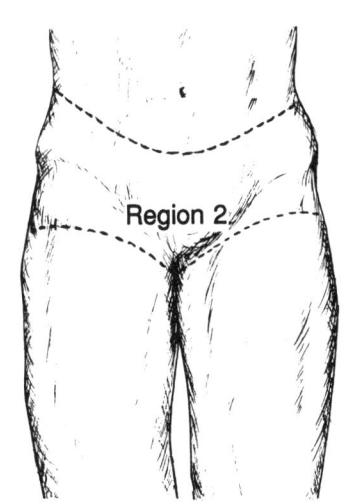

Figure 10–1

The spinal lesion is usually a subluxation that can be classified as primary or secondary, depending upon the status of the tissue involved. It may be found in either an acute or chronic state, recognized as such by the reaction and the condition of the underlying structures. This syndrome refers to two specific pain areas, the iliohypogastric and the ilioinguinal neural regions (see Fig. 10–2).

Either or both these areas may be reactive, but

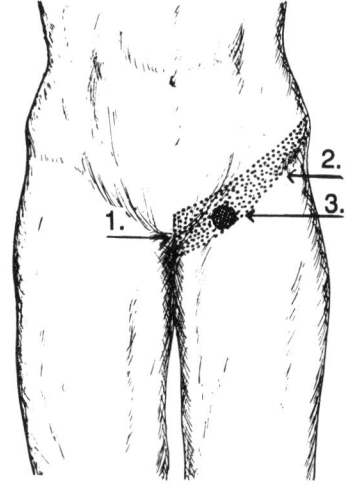

1. Hypogastric Area
2. Inguinal Area
3. Sharpest Pain Area

Figure 10–2

the inguinal area is the most common. The major spinal level involved in this syndrome is the thoracolumbar level and pain is caused by injury from either a primary or secondary lesion to nerve roots arising from the 12th thoracic or the 1st lumbar spinal roots. It is also caused by neural reaction at this level resulting from lesions found lower in the spine, by the shunting of neural impulses from the posterior primary rami to the anterior primary rami.

This pain syndrome is one of three found in the pelvic region and is the only low back/leg pain syndrome on the anterior surface of the body trunk.

Common Areas of Pain Found in This Syndrome

The chief complaint for this condition will be pain at the lower abdomen or along the groin. It is most commonly unilateral, but may occur on both sides in severe lesions.

The inguinal pain syndrome is not difficult for the patient to outline or to indicate small areas of sharp pain within the syndrome area. It is divided into two parts.

1. The first and highest portion is about 2- or 3-inches wide, running parallel to the groin and above it (see Fig. 10–2, #1).
2. The second and lower area is over the groin, extending from the anterior iliac crest to the pubis (see Fig. 10–2, #2). This portion of the inguinal syndrome is the most common, but only in the most severe cases does the pain affect this total area. The sharpest area of pain is most frequently about half way between the iliac crest and the pubis (see Fig. 10–2, #3). In severe cases, the pain is extreme and may extend into the testes in the male or the labia majus in the female. It is often mistaken for a female problem, yet the greatest percentage of cases are found in the male. In severe cases, it is not unusual for the patient to stand in a flexed position because of the extreme pain. It is equally capable of causing total disability. The presence of this pain syndrome often seems to have an emotional effect upon the patient far exceeding all other spinal pain syndromes.

Nerve Supply to This Syndrome Area

The nerve supply to the inguinal pain syndrome is found in the anterior primary rami. The specific nerves are the following.[2]

The upper section (abdominal portion) is supplied from the 12th thoracic nerve and the iliohypogastric nerve. The lower section (groin)[3] is supplied from the iliohypogastric and ilioinguinal nerve. In some cases, the genitofemoral nerve appears to become involved (see Fig. 10–3). This is a minor pain syndrome that may be associated with the inguinal pain syndrome, in rare cases, or it may be present alone. Fibers from this nerve also arise from the 1st lumbar nerve.

Because of individual differences there is considerable anatomical nerve variation found in the lumbar and sacral nerve groups, and these variations might well play a major role in the differences found in pain areas. Anatomical variations are loosely estimated to range from 6% to 12%. Although the inguinal pain syndrome is found in only 4% of all single pain cases, it allows ample latitude.

Characteristics

In order to better understand this syndrome, its present statistics are offered below.

The inguinal syndrome is found in 4% of all single pain syndromes. It is, however, frequently associated with other pain syndromes.

The major spinal joint level of injury or reaction is the 12th thoracic and results from a response or injury to the anterior primary rami. It is found in 60% of male and in 40% female cases. Acute cases appeared in 53%, with the balance of 47%, chronic.

The type of injury is found in the following percentages.

1. Twisting   47%
2. Lifting   13%
3. Bending   7%
4. Fall   1%
5. Struck   7%
6. Unknown   40%

The spinal levels of injury or reaction found by the spinal segmental examination are

1. 12th thoracic   100%
2. 5th lumbar   13%

Spinal levels treated by specific manipulation are

1. 12th thoracic   100%
2. 5th lumbar   13%

Two points found in the statistics regarding this syndrome are of interest and the second seems to differentiate it sharply from other pain syndromes caused by spinal lesions. First, the acute and chronic cases are approximately equal (acute: 53%; chronic: 47%). These figures are quite different from those seen in the paraspinal and lumbar syndromes. It indicates that a large percentage of the acute cases become secondary and chronic lesions. The implication is that ineffective treatment or lack of patient cooperation may be the basis for this syndrome's chronic existence.

The second point is that the greatest percentage of injuries noted for the inguinal pain syndrome

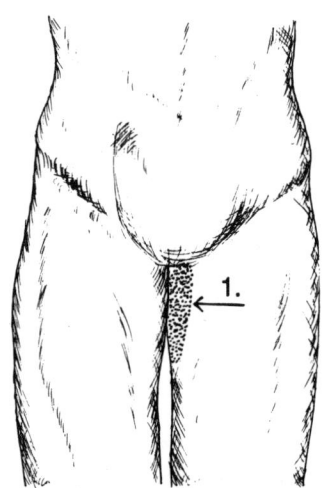

Figure 10–3   1. Genitofemoral Area

are caused by the patient twisting. This particular motion is frequently found a cause of thoracolumbar spinal lesions in low back/leg pain syndromes, and may be the primary reason for most lesions at that area.

Examination Findings for the Inguinal Pain Syndrome

During the author's research into the inguinal syndrome, the spinal segmental examination indicated that every such case was caused by a spinal lesion or reaction found at the thoracolumbar level, most specifically the 12th thoracic segment. The Soto Hall and Linders tests may be positive in some cases, but are not a definitive sign that this condition exists. A secondary spinal lesion at the thoracolumbar junction will be found in most of these cases. Note that in 40% of these cases the patient is unaware of any injury that might be a causative factor.

The complete regional orthopedic examination for this pain syndrome is as important as it is with all low back/leg pain syndromes. Pain from the inguinal syndrome must be differentiated from abdominal, pelvic, hip, and reproductive organ lesions as well as destructive lesions found at spinal levels. Once the doctor is reasonably certain that the condition arises from a spinal lesion, the spinal segmental examination is essential to locate the level of the lesion and it should then be classified as primary or secondary.

DISCUSSION RELATED TO TREATMENT

The response from treatment to the 12th thoracic–1st lumbar level was more than gratifying to those patients who suffered from this difficult pain syndrome. The physician cannot, however, ignore the 13% reaction found at the 5th lumbar spinal level, nor the fact that this level was treated concurrently with the 12th thoracic in those cases when it was present. Because it is known that a direct nerve supply from the 5th lumbar level to the syndrome described does not exist, this area, nevertheless, seems to influence that syndrome; there must be a neurologic connection that links these two.[4] (A hypothesis of how this pain mechanism appears to work is found in the chapter on pain mechanism.)

Injury to the 5th lumbar segment causing a lesion at that motor unit can send neural impulses to the nerve centers at the thoracolumbar level, which control antalgic contraction for spinal protection. Variation of the lumbar plexus may cause a bypass, shunting these impulses to the anterior neural rami, thus causing the inguinal pain syndrome. Flooded with these abnormal neural impulses, the 12th thoracic motor unit becomes reactive; this reaction would be picked up by the spinal segmental examination. This author's first real understanding of the relationship between lesions found at the thoracolumbar level and the linking of these lesions to the inguinal syndrome occurred about 10 years ago. Since that time, many cases have been treated, some single syndromes and many combined with others. Problems are inherent and difficult in its treatment, although this condition, particularly in the acute stage, is rather easy to correct or control. The author feels that these problems create the groundwork for a future chronic condition.

The major problem related to these cases appears to be difficulties in convincing the patient that this pain area is generally a direct result of some type of lesion found at spinal joints. Because of the pain's proximity to abdominal structures and reproductive organs, the patient wants and expects almost immediate relief. This desire seems to stem from fear that the reproductive organs would or could be involved, and might affect sexual performance, or that abdominal organs are involved that might require surgery. When this immediate relief does not appear, another physician is often sought. A round of doctors continues until the patient becomes exhausted and is frequently financially depleted. Because medication does not correct a spinal lesion, some patients ultimately come to the chiropractor. Those chiropractors not familiar with all of the ramifications of these cases often lose them. The consequence is often unnecessary surgery; in any event, the condition frequently becomes chronic. Probably the greatest percentage of inguinal pain syndrome cases have repeated this pattern and are chronically suffering from this condition, which could have been corrected or controlled at an early stage. Cases that are chronic and almost beyond the aid of any form of treatment indicate progressive degeneration at the thoracolumbar spine.

Many patients with these cases come to the office for treatment, not for that condition, but for other spinal pain syndromes. Those patients have lost all hope that anything can be done for chronic pain at the inguinal area. It is unfortunate, because chronic lesions at the thoracolumbar area tend to cause other pain syndromes when they become secondary. It is likely that they will affect neighboring spinal segments.

The acute stage of this pain syndrome appears to last for a long time, usually months, and during that period it can be treated with hope for complete success. When the inguinal pain increases until it becomes severe or becomes static and extends into the testes or labia, causing some forms of disability, particularly in sexual activities, the patient seems to lose all hope and no longer seeks conservative treatment. One of the first signs of a chronic inguinal syndrome is swelling of superficial inguinal lymphatic nodes. A number of patients have one or more surgical procedures because of this syndrome, with little to no benefit. The greatest result in severe cases seems to be the reduction of severe pain to a lesser although chronic pain level.

In a few cases, the pain bypasses the reproductive organs and affects the genitofemoral nerve, causing pain at the upper medial portion of the leg. This does not lessen the effect upon the patient, because slight lateral movements or external rotation of the leg tend to increase the pain. The emotional problems because of the proximity to the reproductive organs are still present.

With background knowledge of this condition, it could be expected that the 12th thoracic lesion is always associated with it, and this may be true. It is not certain that secondary spinal lesions unreactive to the segmental examination and found at any level below the 12th thoracic segment, which might be the primary neural activator in the cause of this syndrome, do not exist.

When the inguinal syndrome results from a secondary lesion found at the thoracolumbar level, it is difficult to resolve, and every effort must be undertaken to control this condition. It appears that ultrasound used bilaterally to the lesion before treatment with specific segmental manipulation is the most effective treatment. Ultrasound to the swollen nodes along the inguinal region also appears to be highly effective. The cause of this condition, a primary or secondary subluxation/disrelation lesion, must be reduced when possible, in order that healing take place at and around the spinal nerve roots.

When a primary lesion is present, the objective of the treatment is correction as soon as possible to prevent it from becoming a secondary lesion. When this condition is a severe secondary spinal lesion, control and the reduction of pain is probably all that can be hoped for. Like many others of the human body, this condition is best prevented or terminated during the acute stage. Those few patients susceptible to this syndrome should be warned during the acute stage that this syndrome is subject to recurrence, and that the spinal lesion frequently becomes secondary. Periodic spinal examination of the thoracolumbar region in these cases is highly recommended.

REFERENCES

1. Thomas JE: Classification of low back/leg pain syndromes, Part 2. *FCA Journal* November–December: p.18, 1985
2. Thomas JE: Classification of low back/leg pain syndromes, Part 3. *FCA Journal* January–February:p.37, 1986
3. Gray H: *Gray's Anatomy,* 30th ed. Philadelphia, Lea & Febiger, 1984;p.1223
4. Thomas JE: Classification of Low Back/Leg Pain Syndromes, Part 5. *FCA Journal* July–August:p.32, 1986

Chapter 11

Thomas Pain Syndrome

One of the most misdiagnosed of the low back/leg pain syndromes caused by spinal lesions is the Thomas syndrome, found in the pelvic region. It overlays the upper and posterior body area near the hip joint extending to areas over the lateral gluteal muscles. Because of this location, it is frequently diagnosed as a hip lesion or a lesion of the lumbosacral joint (see Fig. 11–1).

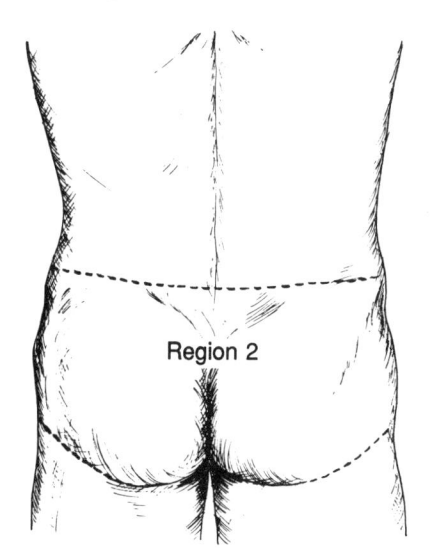

Figure 11–1

THOMAS PAIN SYNDROME

This pain area was the first pain syndrome area outlined by the author in 1975. It overlays the hip joint and posterior surrounding tissue and is divided into two pain areas (see Figs. 11–2 and 11–3).[1,2]

Common Areas of Pain Found in This Syndrome

Pain may be found in this pain syndrome area in two distinct locations. Either location or both may be present in any given case.

1. A small pain area is triangular in shape and lies immediately above the greater trochanter of the femur. It extends upward, and forms a base approximately 2-inches wide at the iliac crest. When activated, this area appears to be the more painful and debilitating of the two areas, but is found less frequently (see #1, Figs. 11–2, 11–3).

2. The second pain area extends immediately behind the smaller one and fans out over the posterolateral gluteus. The base of the thumb should be placed at the iliac crest centerline and the fingers opened or spread backward; this will take in both portions of this pain syndrome fairly well. The second pain area is the more common and is frequently associated with other pain syndromes (see #2, Figs. 11–2, 11–3).

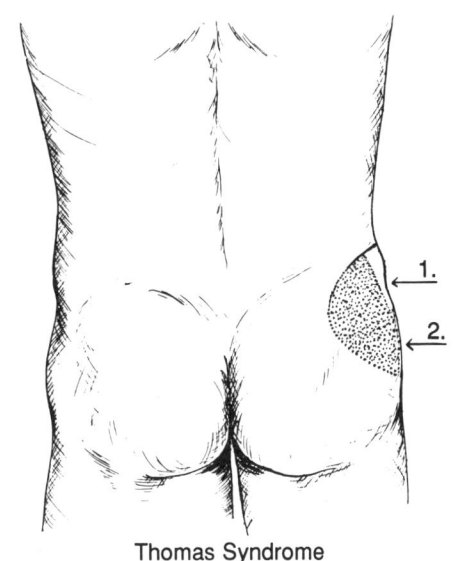

Thomas Syndrome **Figure 11–2**

Nerve Supply for This Syndrome Area

A dual nerve supply, the lateral cutaneous branches of both the 12th thoracic and iliohypogastric nerves, innervate the tissues of this area. The 12th thoracic nerve appears responsible for the smaller pain area found above the trochanter, whereas the posterior portion of this syndrome is

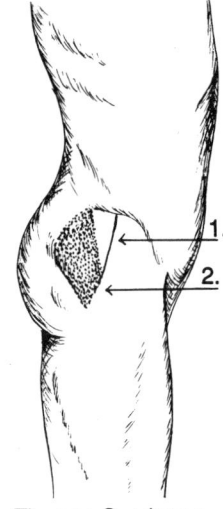

Figure 11-3 Thomas Syndrome

supplied by the iliohypogastric nerve. These nerves may, however, be anatomically inverse in size, or one may be absent, causing variations that may affect the pain syndromes. Because the Thomas syndrome approximates the upper and posterior area of the hip, it is most frequently considered a hip problem, and diagnosed as hip arthritis when no x-ray evidence is seen, nor is there a positive arthritic profile. Many patients with this condition, who have been on arthritic medication, become pain free following specific manipulation to the spinal joint lesions that were the real cause of the problem. This syndrome has individual characteristics, as do other low back/leg pain syndromes, and it is important to become familiar with them.

Characteristics

The Thomas syndrome is found in approximately 4% of all single pain syndrome cases.[4] The major level of injury is found to be the 12th thoracic/1st lumbar spinal level, involving the anterior primary rami. It appears in 60% of females and 40% of males. Acute cases account for 80%, whereas chronic cases are present in 20%.

The types of injuries incurred are found in the following percentages.

1. Lifting   27%
2. Bending   13%
3. Twisting   13%
4. Fall   7%
5. Struck   7%
6. Push–pull   7%
7. Unknown   33%

The spinal levels of injury or reaction are found in the following percentages.

1. 12T   60%
2. 4L   7%
3. 4L & 12T   0%
4. 5L   7%
5. 5L & 12T   20%
6. Other   20%

Totals for each primary levels injured are

1. 12th thoracic   80%
2. 5th lumbar   27%
3. 4th lumbar   7%
4. Other   20%

Spinal level treated by specific manipulation are

1. 12th thoracic   87%
2. 5th lumbar   20%
3. 4th lumbar   7%

Of interest in this syndrome is that lifting, which is second only to unknown causes, seems to be the most predominant injury, and more women than men develop this syndrome. Note that when combined, bending and twisting appear important in the causes of this active syndrome.

When some of the differences in the characteristics of low back/leg pain syndromes are known, a better understanding of all low back/leg pain is provided and, hence, better understanding of the spinal lesion. Lesions found at the thoracolumbar level take precedence for the causes of the paraspinal, inguinal, and Thomas pain syndromes. Neural anatomical variance from patient to patient may well be the reason for the inclusion of either the inguinal or Thomas syndrome, or both, in the pelvic region. Better evidence is needed for certainty.

The 12th thoracic/1st lumbar motor unit appears to be the major spinal unit involved for the paraspinal, inguinal, and Thomas syndromes, as well as being of varying importance in all other low back/leg pain syndromes. As described in Chapter 10, the mechanism of pain would account for that area's activation by lesions found below the 12th thoracic spinal level, but certainly would not explain the different direction these neural impulses take resulting in different syndromes affected. We know that normal anatomical variations in the size of these nerves and in their relationship to one another are found in the lumbar plexus, particularly at the upper portion of that plexus. It is necessary to consider that this anatomical maze may accept neural impulses and distribute those impulses in a fashion not expected nor understood at the present time, especially if the neural tissues are flooded by neural impulses. The anatomical differences that can affect the neural location of some pain syndromes may be no more complicated than the color of a patient's hair or eyes.

During the initial consultation when the chiropractor asks the patient where the pain is located, the usual answer when affected by the Thomas pain syndrome is, "The pain is in my hip." This is the most frequently heard reply when the upper or triangle portion is activated or when small areas of pain are present close to the hip joint and found in the posterior portion of the Thomas syndrome area. When the pain is confined to the posterior portion of this syndrome, the reply is usually a gesture. The patient will place his/her hand over the posterolateral hip much like a man reaching for his wallet, thus indicating, "Here is the area of pain."

Examination Findings for the Thomas Pain Syndrome

The examination for this pain syndrome is the same as that conducted for all low back/leg pain syndromes, but specific emphasis must be placed on the possibility of a hip lesion. The chiropractor should investigate for crepitus, such as found in hip arthritis, and reduction of hip motion in varying directions. The practitioner should not, however, be misled, because the pain involved in this condition does reduce the motion of the hip. X-ray of the hip including x-ray of the low back region is certainly recommended. Once certain that hip and upper femur pathology are not present, the physician can attribute the physical findings to the spinal lesion. The spinal x-rays and the patient history aid in the distinction made between a primary and a secondary spinal lesion. The spinal segmental examination will locate the active segment or segments and will rate their response to testing. The highest reactive segment holds the greatest priority for treatment in most cases.

DISCUSSION RELATED TO TREATMENT

Because the spinal segmental examination findings will be the principal guideline related to the eventual method of treatment for this case, the level, reaction, and classification of the lesion at that level are all important. Cases in which a primary lesion is found at thoracolumbar segments can be resolved following specific spinal segmental manipulation at that level. Ultrasound over the pain areas and bilateral to the lesion help to speed the recovery time. Secondary reactive lesions causing this condition create additional problems, depending upon the type of lesion, its location, and its characteristics. An old subluxation/disrelation injury due to torsion can be treated with some expectation that control is possible. Even a long-standing compression fracture or spondylosis, nonreactive but changing its status to a reactive state following an injury, may become controlled with corrective treatment for the superimposed subluxation/disrelation injury.

In the average patient exhibiting the Thomas pain syndrome, it is to be expected that little is shown during the regional orthopedic examination. There may be some pain over the hip area when the SLR test is conducted. This is not a positive SLR test for the lumbosacral joint, only an observation that muscles around the hip are sensitive to painful and mildly contracted. The results of a Fabere test are positive because rotation of the hip further irritates posterior muscles, particularly when the triangular portion of this syndrome is involved. Depending upon the severity of the lesion, principally during the acute stage, a positive finding might be expected when the Soto Hall or Linders tests are performed. When either of these tests are positive, we can expect a high rating for the spinal segmental examination at the reactive level. A consistent or diagnostic, regional orthopedic examination finding does not exist, with the possible exception of muscle contraction close to the posterior hip. The spinal segmental test findings should always be used as the guide for locating the lesion and grading the severity of the lesion. Palpation above the trochanter of the femur causes an increase in pain in the triangular area mentioned previously, when this region is involved. When painful, the posterior portion of the Thomas syndrome may demonstrate isolated areas of sharp pain upon probing. The use of ultrasound at these painful spots will speed the recovery in these cases.

At first, the spinal specific manipulation should be confined to the most reactive segment shown by the segmental examination. In many cases, this will be the 12th thoracic segment. When this reaction is reduced, and a lower segment that was previously reactive is still reactive, treatment should then be started at that area while continuing to monitor the 12th thoracic/1st lumbar level. Cases in which only the lower segments are reactive should be treated, but it is also important to ensure that no segmental restriction or muscle contraction is found at the thoracolumbar segments; treatment to this level should be highly considered, as the nerve root for the condition lies at that level.

Patients presenting with these cases rarely see the chiropractor first and the condition is frequently diagnosed by the medical physician as hip arthritis regardless of the fact that there is no x-ray evidence or lab findings confirming this state. Many cases seen by the chiropractor will have been treated with some form of arthritic medication. Secondary spinal lesions are commonly found in this condition and are frequently arthritic, degenerative arthritis, loss of disc space, or both; this may account for the arthritic medication recommended. Most of these patients will have unconsciously reduced their movements of the hip, particularly lateral movement. Some form of mild exercise to increase this lateral movement should be recommended. Many of these cases are not easy. The patient should be told that time is required for treatment, and that when these cases are not diagnosed and treated properly, the sequel is hip joint degeneration because of the loss of motion.

REFERENCES

1. Gray H: *Gray's Anatomy,* 30th ed. Philadelphia, Lea & Febiger, 1984;p.1223
2. Hamilton WJ: *Textbook of Human Anatomy,* 2nd ed. St. Louis, MO, CV Mosby Co, 1976;p.639
3. Gray H: *Gray's Anatomy,* 30th ed. Philadelphia, Lea & Febiger, 1984;p.1237
4. Thomas JE: Classification of low back/leg pain syndromes—pain syndromes, Part 4 of a series (Part 2). *FCA Journal* May–June:p.38, 1986

Chapter 12

Gluteal Pain Syndrome

The gluteal pain syndrome is the most difficult for the physician and the patient to understand. It is the only major pain syndrome that arises from the posterior primary neural rami but is found outside of the low-back region, located in the pelvis (see Fig. 12–1).

GLUTEAL PAIN SYNDROME

When no other low back/leg pain syndrome is present, this pain area is very precise, its perimeters easily outlined by the patient. Although not commonly found alone, it meets the criteria for pain syndromes and must be considered such. This syndrome denotes an area about the size of a baseball and is located above and lateral to the ischial tuberosity (see Fig. 12–2).

It is generally quite persistent and very painful. Because sitting is most difficult when this syndrome is present, it can be disastrous for those with occupations requiring sitting for long periods of time. For those patients who must walk as a part of their employment, complaints of pain and leg weakness are common. The leg weakness often tends to remain for a short time even after the pain is gone.

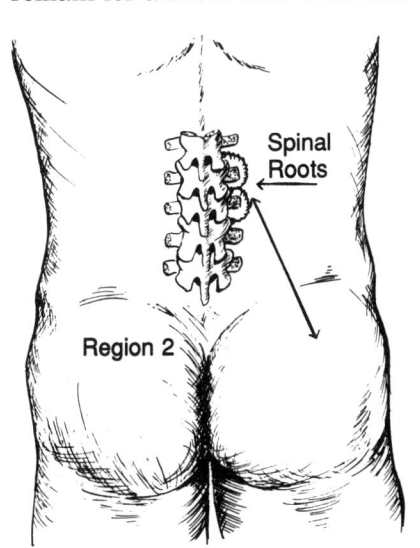

Figure 12–1

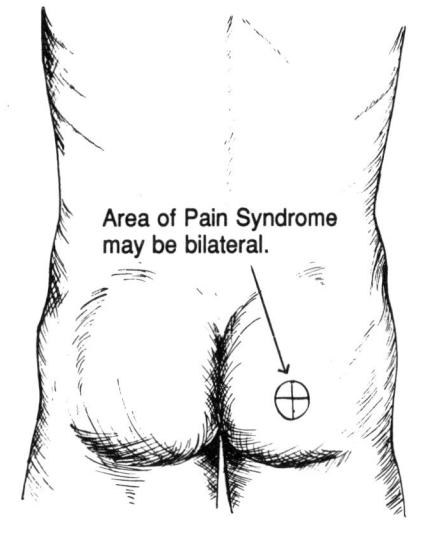

Figure 12–2

Area of Pain Found in This Syndrome

When found as a single pain syndrome, the patient will have no problem pointing to this pain area. He or she can place fingertips precisely over the pain area and will state that no other areas of pain are present. It is most commonly unilateral, but does occur bilaterally.

Nerve Supply to This Syndrome Area

The gluteal pain syndrome appears to be caused by irritation to branches from the superior cluneal nerves.[1,2] These nerves arise from the posterior primary rami with their root level at the 1st, 2nd, and 3rd lumbar, respectively.[3] They extend downward from these levels and innervate the cutaneous area over the gluteal muscles. There is occasionally some underlying tenderness, pain, or both to the gluteal muscles. Aided by upper sacral nerves, nerve fibers from the 4th and 5th lumbar spinal levels innervate the gluteal group. The presence or absence of gluteal muscle pain does not, however, change the pain pattern, nor does the pain appear consistent when the 4th or 5th lumbar nerve is injured. Fibers from the 4th lumbar and possibly from the 5th may, in rare cases, reinforce the cluneal nerves.[4]

Characteristics

The gluteal syndrome is found in only 3% of all single pain syndrome cases and is the smallest pain area statistically acceptable as a major pain syndrome.[5] In most of these cases, the spinal level most commonly reactive is the 12th thoracic (posterior primary rami). It appears to affect the females primarily (55%) and males less so (45%). It is acute in 91%, and 9% become chronic.

The type of injury is found in the following percentages.

1. Lifting   27%
2. Twisting   27%
3. Bending   9%
4. Fall   9%
5. Push–pull   9%
6. Unknown   27%

The spinal levels of injury or reaction found by the spinal segmental examination are

1. 12th thoracic   82%
2. 5th lumbar   18%
3. 4th lumbar   9%

Spinal levels treated by specific manipulation are

1. 12th thoracic   91%
2. 5th lumbar   27%
3. 4th lumbar   27%

This syndrome also has some unusual characteristics that require consideration. First, lifting and twisting are equally found causes of this condition. Once again, the 12th thoracic spinal level and twisting damage are associated. Second, it affects women more frequently than men, although the figures are close. Note that the Thomas syndrome, also found in the pelvic region and arising from the lumbar plexus, affects the female at an even greater percentage than is affected by the gluteal syndrome. The gluteal syndrome becomes chronic in only 9% of the cases when found alone, but is frequently combined with other pain syndromes.

Most important is that the level of the spinal reaction in the greatest percentage is at the 12th thoracic, although the top spinal level for the cluneal nerves is the 1st lumbar. When conducting specific manipulation to the reactive 12th thoracic segment, it becomes apparent that segmental movement often appears to occur at the 1st lumbar level. Locking of the 1st lumbar segment may, in some cases, cause the 12th thoracic neural system to react. The chiropractor should bear in mind that the most reactive spinal segment is the priority segment for treatment until its reaction is reduced; then attention can be turned to the less reactive segment or nerve root levels. If the nerve root spinal level releases following treatment to the reactive level, so much the better. It is interesting to note that the inguinal and Thomas syndromes, caused by lesions from this level, arise from the anterior primary rami, whereas the gluteal syndrome arises from the posterior primary rami. In most cases when the 4th and 5th lumbar levels are reactive, treatment is still required at the 12th thoracic level, coordinated with treatment at the 5th lumbar level. When this syndrome is found alone, it does not appear to be difficult to correct.

Examination Findings for the Gluteal Pain Syndrome

The examination procedures are the same for all low back/leg pain syndromes regardless of how simple they might appear, and that holds true for the gluteal syndrome. With the exception of pain at the gluteal region, there will probably be no other findings for the regional orthopedic examination when conducting the straight leg raising (SLR) test (recorded as positive pain noted over gluteal area only). Should the Soto Hall or the Linders tests be positive, serious joint damage may be indicated.

The findings of the spinal segmental examination will probably show the 12th thoracic or 1st lumbar segment as the most reactive, particularly in cases with a primary lesion present. Secondary lesions may be found at any level, even below the 1st lumbar segment. When lower spinal segments are reactive, neurological flooding often affects the 12th thoracic and 1st lumbar levels, causing the gluteal pain syndrome.

It is also interesting to note that the 4th lumbar is reactive in 9% and the 5th lumbar in 18% of cases, yet treatment is required at both levels in 27%. This is the only pain syndrome in which the 4th lumbar appears to be involved in such a great percentage. This pain syndrome appears to be closely associated with both the lumbar posterior and the sacral anterior primary rami.

DISCUSSION RELATED TO TREATMENT

Treatment is always directed at the most reactive segment first.

The 12th thoracic segment is the principal level to be treated in most gluteal pain syndrome cases, with the lower reactive levels to be considered as the 12th thoracic is reduced in its reactive grade.

Specific segmental manipulation is required at the levels mentioned, and in the proper order. Ultrasound at the gluteal region appears to aid, and seems to be most effective when given at 0.2 to 0.3 watts over a period of about 7 min each session. In highly reactive segmental cases, pulsed diathermy might be used to a greater advantage before the specific manipulation. Chronic cases with hypomobile segments or fixation require a sufficient number of treatments to reduce the active rating and encourage mobilization in those cases in which it is possible.

Because this syndrome is most frequently associated with other pain syndromes, the patient should be advised to continue treatment until full recovery. Although it is true that some doctors might question the presence of this syndrome when overall gluteal pain is present and a known 5th lumbar lesion is evident, one must not ignore this syndrome or fail to thoroughly investigate the upper lumbar segments for even the slightest reaction. The physician must bear in mind that if the patient is taking any type of analgesic, milder reactions to spinal segments may be suppressed. If this condition is ignored or overlooked, it can become chronic, with disastrous results.

REFERENCES

1. Hamilton WJ: *Textbook of Human Anatomy,* 2nd Ed. St. Louis MO, CV Mosby Co, 1976;p.638
2. Gray H: *Gray's Anatomy,* 30th ed. Philadelphia, Lea & Febiger, 1984;p.1195
3. Gray H: *Gray's Anatomy,* 30th ed. Philadelphia, Lea & Febiger, 1984;p.405
4. Hoppenfeld S: *Orthopedic Neurology.* Philadelphia, JB Lippincott, 1977;p.67
5. Thomas JE: Classification of low back/leg pain syndromes—pain syndromes, Part 4 of a series (Part 2). *FCA Journal* May–June:p.38, 1986

Chapter 13

Anterior Femoral Pain Syndrome

The anterior femoral pain syndrome is one of three major pain syndromes found in the leg region that are caused by injury or neural reaction to spinal motor units. These pain syndromes can exist with no associated pain to the low back region because they arise from the anterior primary rami.

ANTERIOR FEMORAL PAIN SYNDROME

The anterior femoral pain syndrome area is found in the leg region. It is innervated by the femoral nerve and arises from the anterior primary rami.

Areas of Pain Found in This Syndrome

The pain syndrome area is well-defined in several reference texts (see Fig. 13–1).[1] It is the anterior portion of the thigh, extending from approximately 2 inches below the inguinal ligament to the knee. Only this area of pain is considered the anterior femoral pain syndrome. Many patients indicate that pain is only in the upper half of the thigh. In a few cases, the patient will indicate pain only just above the knee and care must be taken to separate a knee problem from the anterior femoral nerve irritation, which causes mild muscle contraction to the anterior leg. Occasionally, the pain will wrap around the upper and medial side of the knee and may become extremely painful in some cases. Rarely, the pain may extend over the distribution of the saphenous nerve.

Nerve Supply in This Syndrome Area

The nerve supply in this syndrome extends to include the knee and the lower leg.[2] The portions innervating the knee, leg, or both are not classified as the anterior femoral pain syndrome, even though they are extensions of the same nerve or nerve reaction. Two nerves communicate at the knee, the genitofemoral nerve and branches from the saphenous nerve; they form a minor pain syndrome referred to as the *knee pain syndrome,* caused by a spinal lesion to the femoral nerve. Pain may be found at any area surrounding the patella, but is most commonly found at the medial side of the knee over the knee joint (see Figs. 13–2 and 13–3). The knee syndrome may be present without any other pain to the limb, and may be so severe that walking is difficult or even impossible. Although the knee syndrome is not equivalent to the anterior femoral syndrome, it is part of this neural complex. It is often considered arthritis of the knee and treated as such, with little result. As to the reason for these differences in the

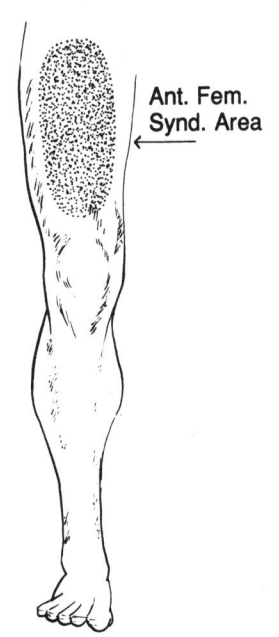

Figure 13–1

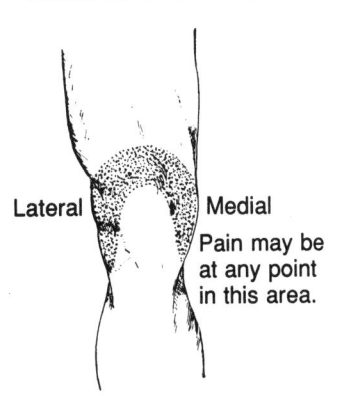

Figure 13–2

Figure 13-3 — Pain Area from Sural Nerve Reaction

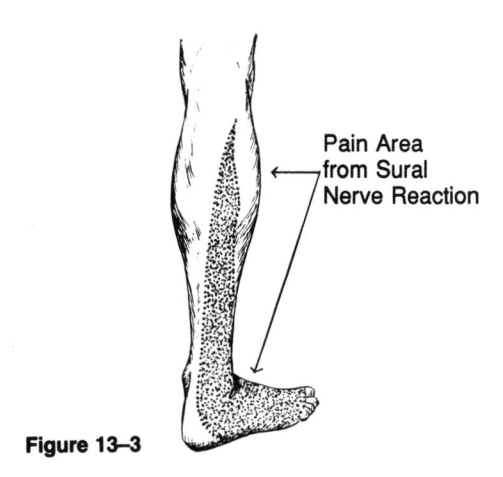

areas of pain, one can only speculate. Perhaps some of these differences are caused by normal anatomical variations found to the neural root. These anatomical variations are not uncommon, as shown by the CAT scan.

A third minor pain syndrome may be present over the saphenous cutaneous nerve distribution. This pain area is occasionally present in the absence of the anterior femoral and knee pain syndromes. When this minor pain syndrome is seen, the pain radiates along the anteromedial portion of the lower leg and extends to the great toe (see Fig. 13-4).

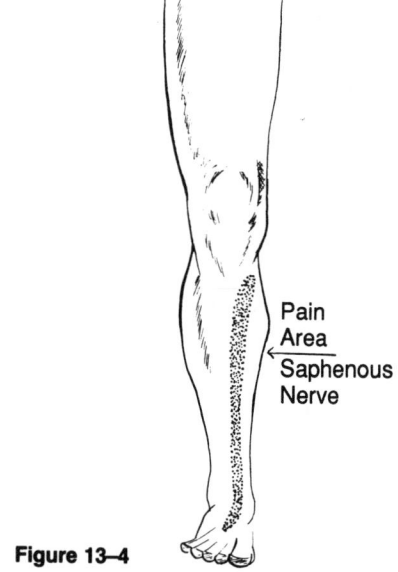

Figure 13-4 — Pain Area Saphenous Nerve

All three pain areas may be present simultaneously, but this is rare. It is found in the most severe cases, and treatment is the same as for the anterior femoral syndrome. Treatment should be continued until all the pain areas are controlled, if possible. When pain is present at the knee or lower medial side of the leg, an examination and possibly x-rays should be considered to eliminate local injury or pathology.

Characteristics

In order to better understand the anterior femoral pain syndrome, its characteristics must be examined.[3]

This syndrome is found in 7% of all single pain syndrome cases; the most commonly reactive major level of injury is the 12th thoracic anterior primary rami. It appears in 55% of male, 45% of female cases. Acute and chronic cases appear to be about equal; acute, 48%; chronic, 52%.

The type of injury is found in the following percentages.

1. Lifting   17%
2. Twisting   21%
3. Bending   17%
4. Fall   7%
5. Push-pull   3%
6. Unknown   52%

The spinal levels of injury or reaction found by the spinal segmental examination are

1. 12th thoracic   100%
2. 5th lumbar   14%
3. 4th lumbar   3%

Spinal levels treated by specific manipulation are

1. 12th thoracic   100%
2. 5th lumbar   10%
3. 4th lumbar   3%

Several points should be considered. The occurrence of this condition is found about equally in both the male and female. It is a condition that is subject to becoming chronic, and the associated pain is often severe enough that the patient has difficulty in walking and even sitting. It is often found in the older patient with secondary lesions such as traumatic or degenerative arthritis, scoliosis, disc thinning, etc. Note that 52% of cases are unable to indicate any accident or injury that precipitated this condition. This finding is incompatible with chronic secondary spinal lesions. Many of the patients who are aware of the condition causing the leg pain indicate that twisting is part of the movement.

Probably most important is the connection between the reactive 12th thoracic segment and this pain syndrome, which is found in every case. Little reaction is shown at other lower spinal segments except the 5th lumbar, which is involved in 14% of cases. It appears that the 5th lumbar reactive lesions are probably secondary lesions rather than a primary cause. It is now known that secondary lesions from the sacral plexus may produce and send a flow of abnormal impulses to the lumbar plexus, involving either the posterior or anterior primary rami. Ten percent of the cases require treatment at the 5th lumbar level in conjunction with the treatment at the 12th thoracic. The chiropractor should always be alert to these connections and reactions, because both levels must be treated although the 12th thoracic in these cases seems to be the primary lesion. Should the 5th lumbar be the most reactive when conducting the spinal segmental examination, it is evaluated as the level of priority for treatment. When the reaction is reduced at that level, the 12th thoracic is then treated, but this reverse reaction is rarely seen.

Examination Findings for the Anterior Femoral Pain Syndrome

Because the 5th lumbar plays a secondary role in most cases of the anterior femoral pain syndrome, a positive straight leg raising (SLR) test (for pain at the 5th lumbar segment) would be found in some cases. Most of these cases, however, produce a negative SLR test. Occasionally, discomfort may be noted over the iliac crest due to the contraction of spinal muscles, resulting from reaction at the thoracolumbar spinal level. A positive Soto Hall or Linders, particularly the Linders, is more realistic. The Fabere test may indicate some discomfort close to the inguinal region or upper portion of the thigh. This is not a positive hip finding, but only the stretching of already painful tissue.

When the minor knee pain syndrome is present, it is wise to examine all tissues of the knee including the patella. The patient can usually place a finger on the exact spot at the lower medial side of the knee. This spot will be over the anteromedial knee joint and is generally the size of a quarter. Occasionally, the patient will indicate discomfort or slight fleeting pains over the anterior thigh, but prime concern is the knee. In those cases in which pain extends down the anteromedial leg to the toe, the patient has no trouble pointing out this area. From time to time, the great toe seems to cause more problems than the leg, and of course investigation of the foot and toe is necessary.

DISCUSSION RELATED TO TREATMENT

Those cases found with a primary spinal lesion are not usually difficult to treat, depending upon the reaction rating found during the spinal segmental examination at the thoracolumbar region, particularly the 12th thoracic segment. High ratings create the most difficulty for treatment at that area. Low ratings can be adjusted by specific segmental manipulation with the patient in a prone position. Pulsed diathermy appears to be most effective when high spinal ratings are found, whereas ultrasound should be used in lower rated cases. Paraspinal muscle contraction seems to lock the spinal segments at reactive levels, reducing motion. It is imperative that this spinal motion be returned to normal when possible to prevent a permanent spinal lesion with its associated pain syndrome, or to prevent additional locking of the secondary lesion.

The use of ultrasound to those pain areas close to the knee is necessary and is effective. When using ultrasound for these lesions, lower wattages for longer periods appear to be the most effective and less apt to cause an increase in pain.

Permanent or secondary spinal lesions at the upper lumbar spinal area appear to be the most common basic cause of most anterior femoral pain syndromes, principally those cases in which the patient is in the geriatric classification, and as a result control of this condition should be uppermost in the chiropractor's mind. The physician should also inform the patient of spinal unit status, indicating the difference between a primary and secondary lesion and that the condition is chronic, should the secondary lesion exist. The patient should be told that periodic treatment may be necessary to continue pain control.

Because the lesion or greatest reaction is found at the 12th thoracic spinal level in all cases of the single anterior femoral pain syndrome, treatment at that level must take priority, even when 5th lumbar reaction is also present as it is in some cases. In double or multiple pain syndromes when the anterior femoral pain syndrome is present, the configuration may be different because of priorities related to the associated pain syndromes. This will be discussed in the chapter on double or multiple pain syndromes.

With rare exception, the anterior femoral pain syndrome is best treated by the conservative method.

REFERENCES

1. Gray H: *Gray's Anatomy,* 30th ed. Philadelphia, Lea & Febiger, 1984;p.1229
2. Hamilton WJ: *Textbook of Human Anatomy,* 2nd ed. St. Louis, CV Mosby Co, 1976;p.659
3. Thomas JE: Classification of low back/leg pain syndromes—pain syndromes, Part 4 of a series (Part 2). *FCA Journal* May–June:p.38, 1986

Chapter 14

Lateral Femoral Pain Syndrome

The lateral femoral pain syndrome is a second pain syndrome found in the leg region, arising from injury or reaction to spinal segments and it results from a reaction of the anterior primary nerve rami.

LATERAL FEMORAL PAIN SYNDROME

The lateral femoral pain syndrome and meralgia parenthetica involve the same cutaneous nerve, with pain found in the same body area. Turek states that it appears that the cause of meralgia parenthetica is unknown, but is thought to be a result of osteoarthritic lesion at the intervertebral foramen.[1] Cailliet feels it is an entrapment of the lateral femoral nerve at the lateral end of the inguinal ligament.[2]

Any nerve pain syndrome can be caused by lesions away from the spine, and such cases would not respond to conservative spinal treatment or any treatment at the spine for that matter. The percentage of cases in this category must be quite small, as all cases in the author's experience with rare exception were caused by spinal lesions. It is always the doctor's responsibility to be alert to the possibility of lesions caused by pain syndromes unassociated with spinal lesions. Knife wounds, loose hip prostheses, tumors, and so on, may be responsible for pain in this syndrome area.

Area of Pain Found in This Syndrome

The lateral femoral pain syndrome refers to an area from the hip to the knee on the lateral side of the thigh[3] (see Fig. 14–1). There are a few cases in which the patient states that pain is present on the side of the leg or crosses below the knee, radiating down the anteromedial side of the leg. A lateral femoral syndrome is still the classification. If both the front and lateral areas of the thigh are painful, a composite is present. Occasionally, the pain is only in the upper half of the lateral femoral pain syndrome area. Like the anterior femoral pain syndrome, this condition can vary considerably in its sensations, ranging from mild discomfort to severe pain. Difficulty in walking and general motion is evident, and the patient may not be free of the pain even in a resting position.

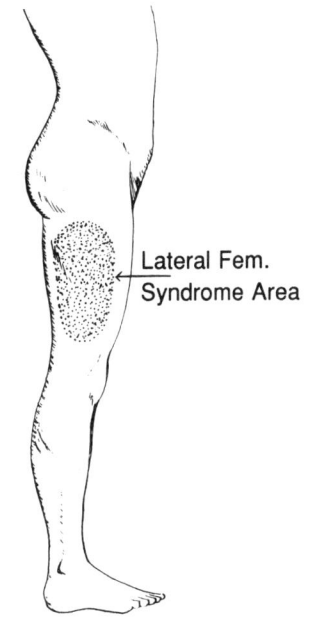

Figure 14–1

Nerve Supply to This Syndrome Area

The nerve supply for the lateral femoral syndrome is the anterior and posterior branches of the lateral femoral cutaneous nerve. This nerve arises from the ventral primary rami found at the 2nd and 3rd lumbar nerve. The anterior branch supplies cutaneous fibers to the anterior and lateral skin of the thigh and ranges down to the knee. The posterior branch supplies the skin from the greater trochanter and the middle of the thigh. The posterior branch appears to be the primary nerve for the lateral pain syndrome, as the area of pain does not extend to the anterior thigh.[4] This nerve also communicates with the saphenous nerve and causes a minor pain syndrome (see Fig. 14–2).

A plexus is formed at the knee by this commu-

Figure 14–2

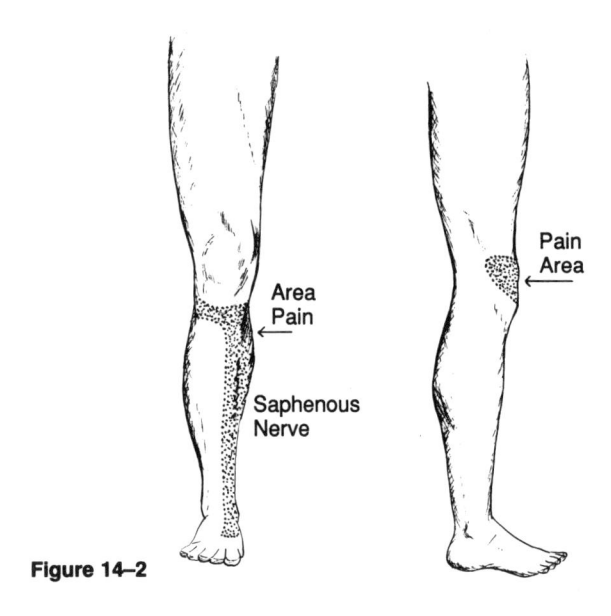

nication and pain can be produced at the medial side of the lower leg to the cutaneous distribution of that nerve. Knee or leg pain is not classified as a part of this syndrome, because it is only present in occasional cases. There must be an awareness of this connection so that when it is present, the doctor is not diverted to some other consideration. The treatment level is not changed.

Characteristics

An investigation of this syndrome's characteristics is necessary for a better understanding of it. The lateral femoral pain syndrome is found in 7% of all single pain syndromes. The most common major level of injury is the 12th thoracic level anterior primary rami. Its effect appears to be equal between the male and female, at 50% each. It also appears to be equal in its status; 50% each of both acute and chronic cases.

The type of injury is found in the following percentages:

1. Lifting 11%
2. Twisting 4%
3. Bending 14%
4. Fall 4%
5. Unknown 75%

The spinal levels of injury or reaction found by the spinal segmental examination are

1. 12th thoracic 92%
2. 5th lumbar 11%
3. 4th lumbar 4%

Spinal levels treated by specific manipulation are

1. 12th thoracic 100%
2. 5th lumbar 14%
3. 4th lumbar 4%

A most important consideration of this syndrome is the fact that 75% of patients have no recollection of an injury or other precipitating cause of their condition. Chronic lesions tend to be present in the greatest percentages of these cases. There is no sex differentiation, both being affected on an equal basis. In considering the spinal levels that are injured or reactive, the 12th thoracic level is once again found to be most reactive, with the 5th lumbar showing a reaction at only 11% of the spinal levels.

Examination Finding for the Lateral Femoral Pain Syndrome

The orthopedic regional examination for this case shows signs similar to that of the anterior femoral syndrome. A straight leg raising (SLR) test will probably be negative in most cases. Because the 5th lumbar segmental rating is shown at only 11%, a positive SLR test may occasionally be found when an old or secondary lesion is present at that level. The doctor should always remember that an old nonreactive lesion (secondary) at any spinal level not producing a pain syndrome may show reaction under testing, but may not be the lesion requiring immediate attention. A lesion with a higher reaction or at the pain syndrome root level always takes precedence. Higher reactive ratings at the 12th thoracic level take precedence over all other spinal levels. Because the pain may be found as high as the hip, the Fabere test may show a positive test. If it is positive, examination or x-rays of the hip are suggested. The Soto Hall or Linders test may be positive if the spinal lesion is highly reactive, or if severe antalgic spasm is present.

Considering the characteristics of this condition, one would expect the 12th thoracic to react to segmental examination in the greatest percentage of these cases, and the statistics verify that it does.

DISCUSSION RELATED TO TREATMENT

The treatment found to be the most effective is specific spinal manipulation, as described for the anterior femoral syndrome. The highest reactive spinal segment is the target for primary treatment. Should it be at the level of the 12th thoracic, that level is treated until the reactive rating is reduced, and then attention is turned to the 2nd and 3rd lumbar root levels; these levels should be followed until the condition is under control or pain free.

Pulsed ultrasound or diathermy can be used before the manipulation process to aid in its effectiveness. Conservative medical treatment has not been effective in this condition, as evidenced by the fact that the impairment rating for the lateral femoral nerve is double the rating of other cutaneous nerves of the leg. This probably indicates that it has been a problem in the diagnosis and treatment.[5]

Under chiropractic care, this condition is no more difficult to diagnose or treat than is the anterior femoral pain syndrome, and the results of the treatment are highly effective.

REFERENCES

1. Turek S: *Orthopaedics:Principles and Their Application,* 3rd ed. Philadelphia, Lippincott, 1959;p.243
2. Cailliet R: *Soft Tissue Pain and Disability*. Philadelphia, FA Davis Co, 1977;p.215
3. Gray H: *Gray's Anatomy,* 30th ed. Philadelphia, Lea & Febiger, 1984;p.1229
4. Gray H: *Gray's Anatomy,* 30th ed. Philadelphia, Lea & Febiger, 1984;p.1229
5. American Medical Association: *Guides to the Evaluation of Permanent Impairment,* 3rd ed. Chicago, American Medical Association, 1988;p.66

Chapter 15

Posterior Femoral Pain Syndrome

Of the eight major pain syndrome areas caused by injury or reaction to tissues found within the spinal joints, the pain area found at the back of the thigh, which occasionally involves the lower leg, without doubt causes the patient and both chiropractic and medical physicians the greatest number of problems of all pain syndromes. It is unfortunate, but the problems associated with this syndrome have for the most part been directly associated with the absence of precise procedures in its diagnosis. There can be no question that cases do occur that are caused by disc lesions or other gross and serious pathology, but the greatest percentage of posterior leg pain has not been found to fall within that category.

POSTERIOR FEMORAL PAIN SYNDROME

In the investigation of posterior leg pain cases, too much emphasis has been placed upon the great sciatic nerve and little or no thought given to the small sciatic nerve, the posterior femoral. This nerve supplies tissue that overlay the great sciatic nerve and it is also subject to reaction[1,2] (see Fig. 15–1). Without a careful diagnostic procedure, these two nerves, which may be the cause of pain, cannot be differentiated.

The two principal causes of sciatica are the fragmented or a grossly bulging disc, causing a direct or indirect pressure on the sciatic nerve root and stenosis that severely reduces the foramenal space occupied by that nerve. The author's statistical research over a period of 25 years has shown that when present, these two factors, particularly disc involvement, also cause a reaction to the posterior primary rami. This can be determined by both the regional and the segmental examination. The findings, by both test procedures, are positive. Even today with the CAT scan and the MRI, it has not been proven by visual evidence that the bulk of posterior leg pain cases are related to the disc lesion, stenosis, or both.

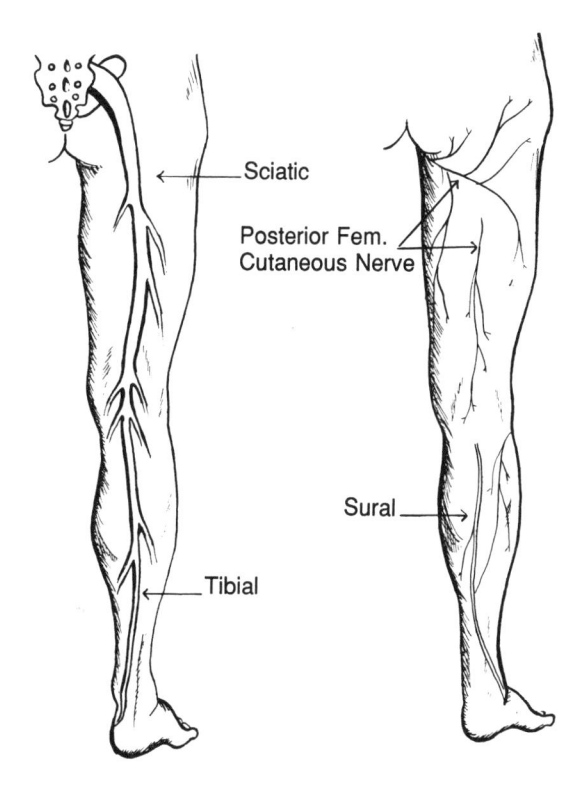

Figure 15–1

Injuries and other pathologies found at the 4th and 5th lumbar spinal levels are only one cause of low back/leg pain syndromes. Studies have shown that individual pain syndromes can be caused from injury or reaction to other spinal levels, even in the absence of 4th and 5th lumbar reactive lesions.[3] The role that lumbosacral lesions play in low back/leg pain syndromes is complex, and several avenues must be considered when they are present. In order to understand this problem, it was necessary to determine the principal pain produced by lesions to this spinal level, and the frequency this level appeared to be injured or reactive. Once this information was known, it was then correlated with all known pain syndromes.

Areas of Pain Found in This Syndrome

The posterior femoral pain syndrome refers to an

area from the base of the buttocks to the back of the knee, over the posterior portion of the thigh[4] (see Fig. 15–2). Pain is not always found in the entire area. Probably the most common area is the upper one half of the posterior thigh. Occasionally, the lower area is the only area involved and in some cases the pain is found only close to the back of the knee.

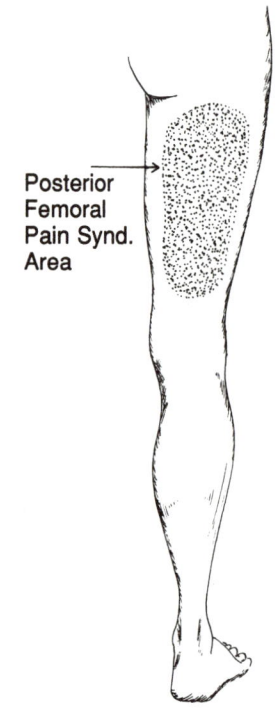

Figure 15–2

Nerve Supply to This Syndrome Area
There are two nerves that may cause pain to the posterior portion of the leg, the posterior femoral nerve and the sciatic nerve.[5] Both these nerves arise from the anterior primary rami.

1. The posterior femoral nerve is a cutaneous nerve and its distribution is that area within the posterior femoral pain syndrome area designated by the back of the thigh. In some cases, the pain extends down the posterolateral portion of the lower leg to the little toe (see Fig. 15–3). This extended pain area constitutes another minor pain syndrome. The nerve involved is the sural nerve and it communicates with the posterior femoral nerve. On occasion, it may be the only pain area present. One might wonder why pain would bypass the posterior femoral or sciatic nerve to produce pain to the lower leg; again, differences in anatomical neural linkage at the nerve roots may be the differential factor.
2. The sciatic nerve is a deep nerve also found at the posterior portion of the upper thigh. Its pain areas are similar to the posterior femoral nerve.

It is a major nerve and highly subject to pain caused by the bulging or fragmentation of a vertebral disc, stenosis, or both. Its reaction appears in less than 3% of cases and is, therefore, not listed as a primary pain syndrome, regardless of the fact that, when reactive, it constitutes a major problem. The pain syndromes are not recorded according to their severity, but their frequency.

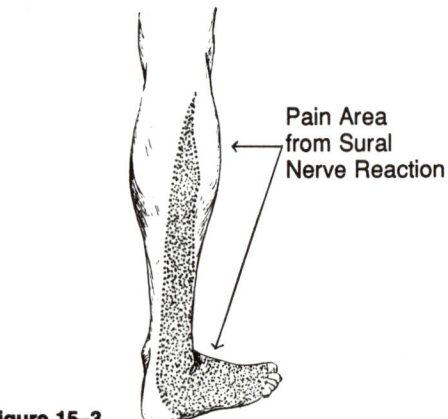

Figure 15–3

Characteristics
The posterior femoral pain syndrome is found in only 6% of all single pain syndrome cases and is a result of reaction from the anterior primary rami. The most common major level of injury or reaction is found to be the 5th lumbar. It appears in 56% of males, and with 44% of females. It is acute in 56%, and chronic in 44%.

The types of injury are found in the following percentages:

1.	Lifting	11%
2.	Twisting	22%
3.	Bending	22%
4.	Fall	11%
5.	Struck	7%
6.	Unknown	48%

The spinal levels of injury or reaction found by the spinal segmental examination are

1.	12th thoracic	52%
2.	5th lumbar	62%
3.	4th lumbar	11%

Spinal levels treated by specific manipulation are

1.	12th thoracic	56%
2.	5th lumbar	74%
3.	4th lumbar	7%

There is no great difference between the number of cases found in males and females. The number of chronic cases is close to the number of acute cases. This is never a good sign, as it indicates that current evaluation and treatment of these cases are losing the battle in its control. Of the cases, 48% are unable to determine an injury that might be related to the cause of pain. The greatest number of patients aware of an injury or motion state that twisting while bending was the cause. Lifting does not seem to play a major role in these cases because it is found in only 11% of cases.

The most startling information about this pain syndrome is that only 6% are found in all single pain syndrome cases. Cases of true disc lesions as causation factors of sciatic compression at the fifth lumbar level were not in sufficient numbers to be classified; because the author's lowest statistical classification for single low back/leg pain syndromes was 3%, this condition was not considered a major pain syndrome. Although it is true that even one disc lesion directly responsible for leg pain is important, the correct diagnosis for posterior leg pain is more important.

Equally surprising are the figures for spinal injury and reaction in this syndrome. With the presence of the posterior pain syndrome, the 5th lumbar motor unit is reactive to examination in only 62% of these cases. Even when combined with the 4th lumbar unit, the total is only 73%. This leaves a minimum of 27% of posterior femoral pain syndromes not showing a reactive rating at either the 4th or 5th lumbar segment. It also indicates that low-grade lesions can be present, nonreactive to examination, but still capable of producing neural reaction sufficient to cause the posterior femoral pain syndrome.

The presence of a 12th thoracic reactive lesion combined with this syndrome in 56% of the cases was certainly not anticipated during the clinical research, as this combination follows the pattern found in all other leg pain syndromes. The difference is that the neural levels in other leg syndromes are from the lumbar plexus, whereas this syndrome arises from the sacral plexus. It was felt that this might make a difference. It shows that the pain syndromes of lumbar plexus lesions are in many cases related to the 12th thoracic spinal levels. They are probably the cause of 12th thoracic reactive lesions and pain syndromes from that level.

The doctor questions how it can be ascertained that the 12th thoracic reactive segment is not from a previous injury at that level rather than the 5th lumbar? This is a valid question and can be answered only one way. It cannot be. There are, however, certain points that may be considered. First, no pain syndromes arising from the thoracolumbar region are present in these cases. Second, with that great a percentage of injuries occurring at the 12th thoracic region in posterior leg pain cases, it is necessary to ask if that lesion is responsible in some way for the 5th lumbar lesion? The author does not feel it functions in that way, but the question remains. Another important indication is that treatment to the most reactive segment takes priority over all others. In those composite pain syndrome cases when the 12th thoracic is most reactive, treatment at that area often reduces the posterior leg pain even before the 5th lumbar is treated. In cases when no reaction is found at the 5th lumbar level, but reaction occurs at the 12th thoracic, treatment at that level often terminates the leg pain without treatment to the 5th lumbar level. More recent work related to this problem points to the possibility that muscle antalgic contraction at the 4th and 5th lumbar segments, compressing or immobilizing the joint caused by lesions above this level, may produce irritation to the sciatic nerve. One could, of course, speculate about this for some time and nevertheless not know all the answers, or even all of the questions.

It is important, however, that an increase in knowledge regarding this pain syndrome has been gained, and with the use of this knowledge can gain still more.

Examination Findings for the Posterior Femoral Pain Syndrome

When a case of posterior femoral pain is examined, the interpretation of the findings is important and must be consistent. When the straight leg raising (SLR) test is conducted, a reactive 5th lumbar lesion produces a positive finding. For a positive SLR test, the pain must reside immediately over the lumbosacral joint. (**No other area is acceptable as positive for a 5th lumbar lesion.**) Secondary lesions are often present as low-grade nonreactive lesions, and the SLR test is frequently negative in those cases. There may be no difference in the intensity of the posterior leg pain between these two classifications of the lesion. Depending upon the lesion, there may be either a positive or negative finding at the 5th lumbar level. The purpose for these tests is to determine the status of the spinal lesion.

One is known to exist because the pain syndrome is present. During the leg raising, if severe posterior leg pain is apparent, the leg should be lowered until the pain is reduced, and the ankle should be hyperflexed. If the severe pain returns, it is possible that sciatic pain is present. (Tight or contracted posterior leg muscles should not be confused with sciatic pain.)

The Soto Hall and Linders might be positive or negative depending upon the severity and extent of the lesion; disc lesions at this joint have a positive Linders. One expects the Fabere to be negative unless a hip lesion is also present.

The patient should sit with legs dangling off the table, hands on the lap, and the body erect, not leaning backward. He or she should straighten each leg independently and then both together. This test is almost impossible for a patient with sciatic neuritis.

Spinal segmental examination findings can vary depending upon the extent of the injured tissue and the status of the lesion. Because there is a backlog of information regarding the posterior femoral syndrome, it is known that the 4th and particularly the 5th lumbar are reactive in the greatest percentage of the cases. Case history and x-rays help determine if this area contains a primary or secondary lesion. It is expected that joint reaction will be related to joint status. Because this pain syndrome is a single one, with no back pain present, the doctor need not be concerned that reaction of the posterior primary rami will cause extensive muscle contraction. When the 12th thoracic is reactive, neural impulses from the 5th lumbar to the 12th thoracic have begun, and the rating at the 12th thoracic is usually a good indicator as to the level of 5th lumbar neural reaction. The physician should always keep in mind that the examination findings are indicators for lesion reaction. Reexamination can be conducted in a week, 2 weeks, or a month, when comparison of the findings will provide an accurate update as to treatment results.

A primary lesion will almost always produce a reaction at the joint injured because the injury is to normal tissue. The reaction is usually within the higher limits. When a secondary lesion is reactive due to injury, the rating can vary from mild to severe depending upon the ability of the existing pathological tissue to react. When posterior femoral pain is present, joint reaction to testing at the 5th lumbar unit is usually found. If spinal splinting is present, the 4th lumbar unit will probably react to a lesser degree, and muscles extending over the sacrum are often tender on probing. If seen soon after the injury, primary lesions at the 5th lumbar do not usually demonstrate an associated 12th thoracic reaction. This combination is often found in secondary lesions at the 5th lumbar, particularly when there is a delay of several days in the treatment for primary lesions. It appears that the reaction at the 12th thoracic is caused by neural impulses from the lower lesion, involving the anterior primary rami, which causes a reaction to the posterior primary rami, thus resulting in increased muscle contraction and splinting.

It has been indicated in previous chapters that a disc lesion may be present, but that the disc has no nerve supply, and that the motor unit may be nonreactive related to disc degeneration, bulging, and even fragmentation. Sciatic neuritis or neuralgia can be caused by indirect or direct pressure associated with a disc lesion. To diagnose sciatic neuritis or neuralgia resulting from gross pressure due to a disc lesion, certain tests should be positive with no exceptions. First, the SLR test should be positive with pain immediately over the lumbosacral joint. This indicates that movement at the joint is painful due to some form of nerve root injury or muscle contraction (to protect the motor unit). Second, Bragard's sign should be positive due to a hypersensitive nerve reacting to stretch, and the pain should extend throughout the length of the sciatic nerve. Third, probing along the course of the sciatic nerve should cause sharp pain. Both legs should be examined for comparison. In addition, it is necessary that findings from the spinal segmental examination of the 4th and 5th lumbar units be found within the higher reactive range. Reactive segments not at these two levels cannot be considered confirmation of a disc lesion.

These basic tests are the minimum requirement. A positive Kemp sign and a positive Dejerine's Triad provides added information as to the motor unit status. The CAT scan should be required if the diagnosis of a disc lesion is to be given, otherwise the diagnosis might better be a "possible" or "probable" disc lesion. The CAT scan must confirm the disc lesion at the 4th or 5th lumbar level (or at both); any other level showing pathology is unacceptable for disc involvement at these joints.

These requirements for the diagnosis that a disc lesion is causing either joint or nerve reaction may appear rather rigid, but disc lesions may be present without causing these reactions. Without spinal joint tests, neurological tests to the legs indicate that a nerve is involved, but do not confirm that the primary spinal lesion causing these nerve changes is a disc lesion. Neurological tests aid in determining the extent of nerve pathology whether it is caused by a subluxation lesion, or one of its components such as the disc lesion, stenosis, facet injury, demyelination, nonspecific inflammation, or other neural disease.

No single test can give the answers needed for the evaluation of a case. When the examination procedure is conducted in exactly the same way for all low back/leg pain cases and all possible structures are observed, the examiner is then able to refer and relate the current findings to these data. The information acquired and utilized is just as effective in low back/leg pain cases as it is in any other pathological lesion found within the body.

DISCUSSION RELATED TO TREATMENT

In most cases, when the patient indicates that he or she has pain down the back of the leg, the examining physician's first thought is that a sciatic pain syndrome is present. Most diagnostic problems begin at that point.

Pain produced to the leg from a spinal lesion may arise from either nerve, the sciatic or the posterior femoral, without separate recognition, because the pain area is the same. The severity of the lesion appears, however, to be quite different, and it makes the differential diagnosis between these nerves important. If the primary cause of true sciatic pain is a disc lesion, pressure from disc material is the direct cause of pain. Secondary antalgic reaction follows, in addition to the neural reaction. In the posterior femoral syndrome, gross mechanical pressure does not appear to be a factor and subtle differences can be detected by careful examination. To label the patient as a disc case with associated sciatic neuritis when in fact that patient may have a posterior femoral pain syndrome caused by a lesser spinal lesion, carries a major impact to the patient. The effect on his or her occupation, recreation, and relationship with other individuals might be extensive, as also the difference in overall costs, or the possibility of unnecessary surgery for a lesser condition.

Injury to a nerve root may be caused by many factors without involvement of the disc—soft tissue trauma from repeated strain, microtrauma, injury from changes in adjacent tissue, contraction, and probably the most common, the subluxation/disrelation lesion found at the 5th lumbar. These injuries and tissue changes may cause mild to severe reaction to the nerve root and thus pain.[6]

Many tissues of the pelvis and leg region are supplied by fibers from the 5th lumbar nerve root. The gluteal maximus, obturator, and gemellus muscles are in close proximity to the posterior femoral nerve and they receive fibers from the 5th lumbar root. It may be possible that these muscles and their nerve fibers play a part in causes of posterior femoral pain.

It is also well-known that when injured, nerve fibers react at adjacent spinal levels.[7-9] This metamerism is probably the primary cause of the posterior femoral pain.

Probably the most important consideration in the treatment of the 4th or 5th lumbar joint is that closely associated muscle contraction reduces motion to these joints including the sacrum. Any attempt to adjust the lumbosacral joint without first reducing some of this muscle contraction may be met with failure, increased pain, or both, as well as an increase in the muscle contraction.

It is impossible to discuss every situation that might be present related to pathology of this joint and its reaction, even when it is the single pain syndrome. The muscle antalgic contraction in these cases is local, indicating that short deep spinal muscles are involved but not producing pain; otherwise, the lumbar syndrome would be present. Depending upon the type of lesion and the severity, either diathermy, ultrasound, or both should preceed the specific manipulation. Diathermy over the pain area and ultrasound to the joint is most effective. The side-posture position first treated is always in the same direction that the spinous process has rotated. When examining the patient in the prone position, it is necessary to determine in which direction the spinous process has rotated. For example, if the spinous has rotated to the right, the patient must be first treated lying on the left side. This appears contrary to logic, but the rebound from the adjustment seems to have a greater chance of repositioning the segment than does an attempt to pull the segment against contracted muscles. A thrust to the 5th lumbar, either lateral or headward, is not advisable. The direction of pull is lateral and footward. This procedure is discussed in Chapter 18. If movement occurs, the patient can then be treated from the other side, pulling the spinous into the direction desired, with the finger tips. This may not be possible until after some treatment is given in the prime or first position.

When a paraspinal pain syndrome is present with this syndrome, it is essential that upper spinal segments first be treated to reduce the paraspinal muscle contraction. If this procedure is followed, the lumbosacral joint responds to treatment more easily, with less pain to the patient and with a reduced amount of subsequent muscle soreness.

If present with this syndrome, lumbar pain complicates the treatment. Either diathermy, ultrasound, or both should first be used to the joint. If this equipment is not available, the patient must lie in the side-posture position that is subject to initial treatment for a few minutes to aid in relaxation. The upper leg is propped with a pillow, if necessary. After some relaxation, the physician proceeds as discussed above.

The doctor should always consider the associated paraspinal muscle contraction first in the treatment of any spinal lesion, regardless of its level and try if possible to encourage rather than attempt to violate the contracted muscles.

REFERENCES

1. Gray H: *Gray's Anatomy,* 30th ed. Philadelphia, Lea & Febiger, 1984;p.1236
2. Dvorak J, Dvorak V: *Manual Medicine.* Stuttgart-New York, Thieme-Stratton Inc, 1984;p.65
3. Thomas JE: Classification of low back/leg pain syndromes—pain syndromes, Part 5. *FCA Journal* July-August:32, 1986
4. Hamilton WJ: *Textbook of Human Anatomy,* 2nd ed. St. Louis MO, CV Mosby Co, 1976;p.665
5. Gray H: *Gray's Anatomy,* 30th ed. Philadelphia, Lea & Febiger, 1984;p.1237
6. Rydevik B, Brown M, Lundborg G: Pathoanatomy and pathophysiology of nerve root compression. *Spine* 9(1):7, 1984
7. Best CH, Taylor NB: *The Physiological Basis of Medical Practice,* 4th ed. Baltimore, Williams & Wilkins, 1945;p.847
8. Turek S: *Orthopaedics:Principles and Their Application,* 3rd ed. Philadelphia, JB Lippincott, 1959;p.223
9. Hoppenfeld S: *Orthopedic Neurology.* Philadelphia, JB Lippincott, 1977;p.67

Chapter 16

Composite Pain Syndromes

It has been repeatedly stated in this manual that the chiropractor must understand the characteristics of single pain syndromes. He or she must also have knowledge related to the spinal level of the lesions, both actual and reactive, causing these pain syndromes and the difference between primary and secondary lesions—how they react and how to determine their reaction. The chiropractic physician should be aware that the presence of gross spinal pathology does not necessarily indicate a causation of the patient's pain syndrome unless the spinal segment at that neural root level is reactive to the segmental examination. Without this knowledge, the physician's effectiveness is reduced in resolving the problem.

When dealing with injuries subject to third party involvement, it is important to inform the third party that more than one nerve or nerve group is injured when double or multiple pain syndromes are present. This information can justify necessary treatment that may extend beyond their expectations. It also adds information related to the objective and subjective symptoms suffered by the patient.

COMPOSITE PAIN SYNDROMES

Spinal lesions fall into the two main classifications, primary (initial lesions) or secondary (old, or chronic lesions). Severe injuries can occur to more than one level of the spine, causing multiple primary lesions, thus resulting in double or multiple pain syndromes. A typical example is the young person with multiple spinal injuries from an automobile accident. It appears, however, that most multiple pain syndromes are the result of secondary spinal lesions that have been reinjured. In many cases, a primary lesion may also be associated with the secondary lesion. It is likely that patients ages 45 and up will have secondary spinal lesions for many other reasons: types of occupational injuries, previous personal injuries, birth defects that become reactive, acquired spinal changes, constitutional diseases affecting bone and joints, etc. The segregation of primary and secondary spinal lesions is important when the treatment program is initiated; this consideration will probably surface when third-party payors become involved in the case and litigation becomes imminent.

The examination procedures are designed to determine causes and spinal levels of single pain syndromes; from that determination, an awareness of the varied forces and reactions that take place to create the double and multiple pain syndrome cases follows. By comprehending the reactive and protective mechanism of the spine and its components and using this information in the evaluation of low back/leg pain cases, the ability to differentiate these cases regardless of their complexity is increased.

Composite low back, pelvic, and leg pain syndromes include doubles, those cases with two pain syndromes, and multiples, those cases with three or more pain syndromes. The presence of composite pain syndromes generally indicates that the patient suffers with one or more secondary spinal lesions.

Composite syndromes account for approximately 27% of the doctor's case load related to the total number of low back, pelvic, and leg pain patients. Of that 27%, 21% of the patients have double pain syndromes, and the balance of 6% have 3 or more.

The following combinations appear to be the most frequent.

1. Combined lumbar and paraspinal pain syndromes are found in 10% of the 27% group.
2. The anterior femoral with one other pain syndrome is found in 23% of that group.
3. The lateral femoral syndrome with one other is found in 14% of that group.
4. The posterior femoral with one other syndrome is found in 16% of that group.
5. The final 20% do not appear in any apparent specific combination.

Of greatest importance is that the posterior femoral pain syndrome, combined with one or more other pain syndromes, is only found in a small percentage of the 27% group. Combined with the number found in single pain syndromes, this figure shows that pain found down the back of the leg, involving either the sciatic or posterior femoral nerve, is not one of the more prevalent low back, pelvic, and leg pain conditions. This does not indicate that its presence is of less importance, but it does put the posterior femoral pain syndrome in its proper perspective. It also shows that the overall involvement of the sacral plexus is less than the general consensus. This knowledge should serve as a guide, indicating extra precaution to be observed in the examination and diagnosis of lumbosacral plexus lesions, and primarily that of the lumbar plexus. The chiropractor does not look forward to a patient's presenting symptoms of pain in the back, groin, hip, buttock, and down the leg, but this case scenario happens and the condition must be treated. Without an understanding of the individual pain syndromes, it is easy to lose sight of the spinal level or levels that may be injured or reactive when a patient is suffering from two or more simultaneous pain syndromes. The physician may also be unaware of the individual nerve or nerve groups involved in those lesions, thus resulting in a disorganized treatment procedure. This causes longer periods of suffering for the patient, increased overall costs, greater lost time, and possibly a dissatisfied patient.

The initial isolation of each pain syndrome shows the primary nerve division involved for that case; it also indicates the nerve or nerve groups associated with that pain syndrome, and this information leads to the spinal level where those nerves or nerve groups arise. In composite pain syndromes, both nerve divisions are usually involved, but not always. The regional orthopedic examination indicates the reaction of the tissues that are most important. The follow-up spinal segmental examination locates the reactive spinal segments and rates those segments, providing a guideline for the levels to treat and an indication as to the type and frequency of treatment.

The lumbosacral plexus can no longer be considered a single unit when dealing with low back/leg pain syndromes. It must be divided into the lumbar and sacral plexuses, respectively, and considered only with those pain syndromes that are neurologically affiliated with each plexus. There are two major pain syndromes resulting from injury or reaction to spinal levels carrying sacral plexus nerves. They are the lumbar and the posterior femoral pain syndromes. The paraspinal, gluteal, inguinal, Thomas, anterior femoral, and lateral femoral pain syndromes arise from nerves found within the lumbar plexus. Both the lumbar and sacral plexus nerves are also divided by the anterior and posterior primary neural rami. Each rami or division carries certain primary pain syndromes, found in the above group, as follows.

Injury or reaction to the anterior and posterior primary rami causes pain syndromes at certain general levels. Spinal nerves and their spinal levels have been shown in previous chapters, but it is appropriate to show the anterior and posterior rami nerves once more (see Figs. 16–1 and 16–2).

12th Thoracic/1st Lumbar

Thomas syndrome	Anterior primary rami
Inguinal syndrome	Anterior primary rami
Paraspinal syndrome	Local and away from the spine—posterior primary rami, but confined to the back region

2nd and 3rd Lumbar

Anterior femoral syndrome	Anterior primary rami
Lateral femoral syndrome	Anterior primary rami
Paraspinal syndrome	Local—posterior primary rami
Gluteal syndrome	Posterior primary rami

4th and 5th Lumbar

Posterior femoral syndrome	Anterior primary rami
Lumbar syndrome	Local—including sacrum; posterior primary rami
Posterior primary rami (at 4th, 5th lumbar and sacral levels)	Pain will be local, extend over portions of the sacrum, and may radiate lateral to the sacrum

The above configuration alerts the chiropractor to the general spinal levels that are involved neurologically by giving a neural reference point. The spinal segmental examination indicates the reactive

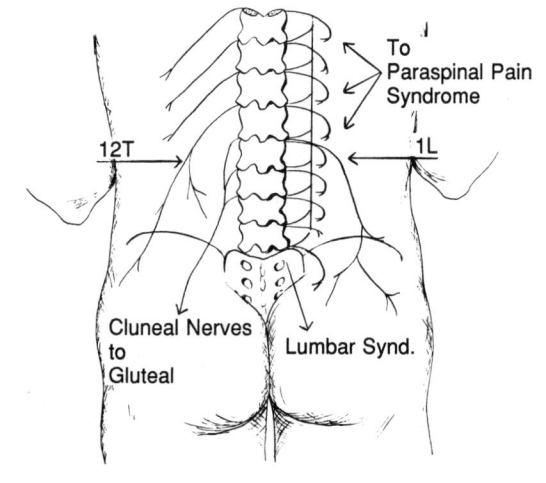

Figure 16–1

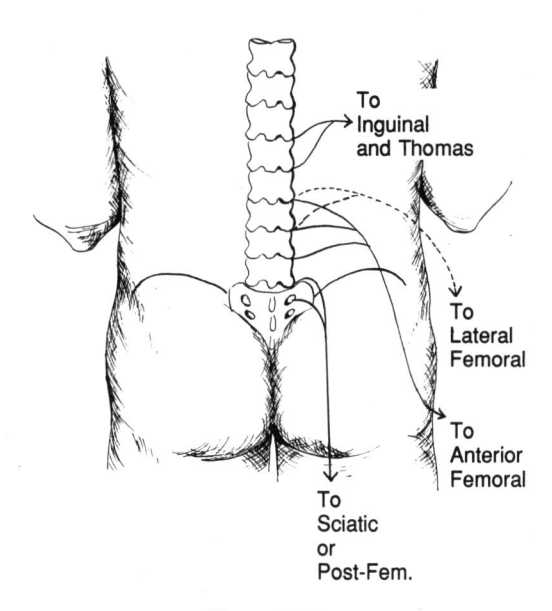

Figure 16-2

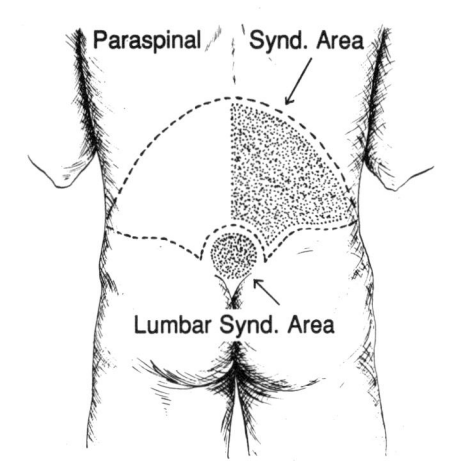

Figure 16-3

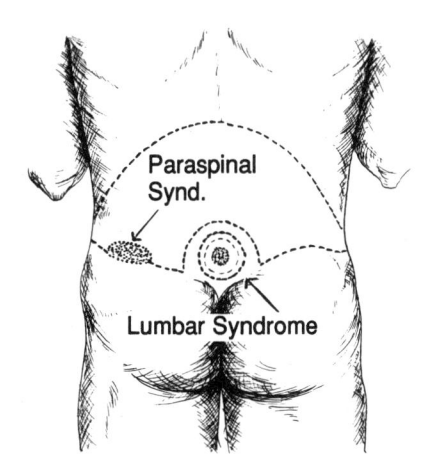

Figure 16-4

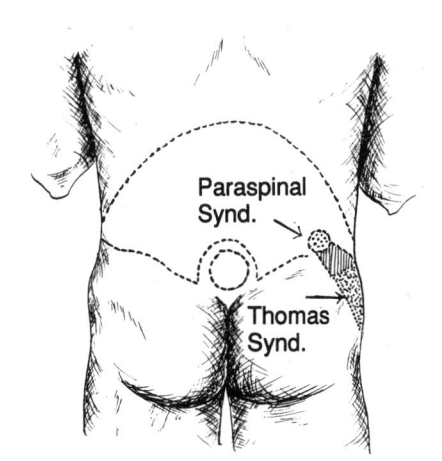

Figure 16-5

rating of each spinal level and points to the area that requires medical attention, as it is the area of physiological reaction.

When the mechanism of pain is understood, and with the knowledge of the individual pain syndromes arising from each level, there should be no difficulty relating to double or multiple pain syndromes. The doctor should always be aware that the anterior and primary rami may react either independently or together under certain circumstances. In some cases, the reasons for this interchange is not fully understood. It is known that an individual anterior primary pain syndrome, such as the inguinal, femoral, and so on, can be present without the posterior primary paraspinal pain syndrome, although the 12th thoracic/1st lumbar segment or segments are reactive to examination, indicating local segmental tissue reaction. It appears that, during the acute stage, the paraspinal pain syndrome is usually present when this segmental reaction is noted, but may in some chronic cases tend to diminish in intensity, and in others to even disappear. Tissue that has changed due to continued injury, neural reaction, or both, appears to respond differently from normal tissue with an acute reaction. This seems to account for many chronic cases of pain syndromes arising from the anterior primary rami when posterior primary pain syndromes are absent.

Before continuing, the various doubles and multiple syndrome cases found in the following figures are presented. Many more could be printed, particularly the multiple pain syndromes (three or more). Figure 16-3 shows the entire paraspinal and lumbar pain syndrome areas as a reference (see Figs. 16-4 through 16-18). (Note that most

Figure 16-6

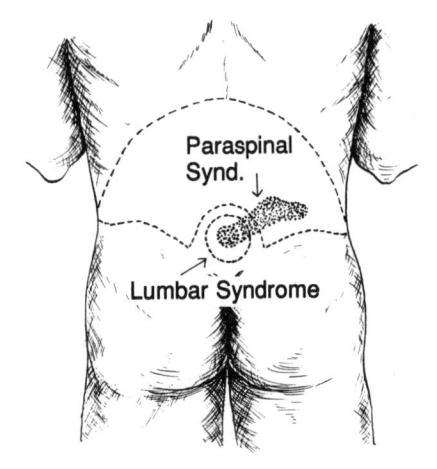

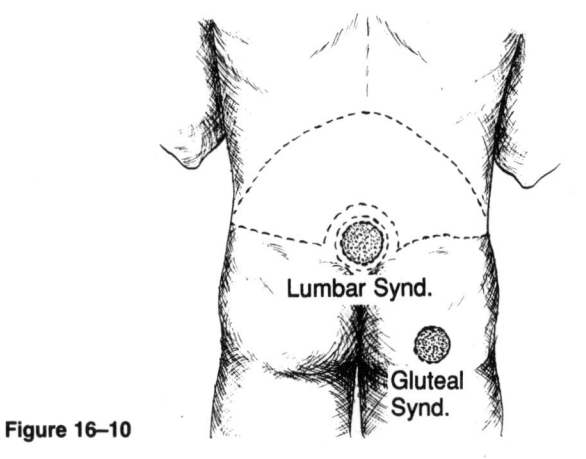

Figure 16-7

Figure 16-8

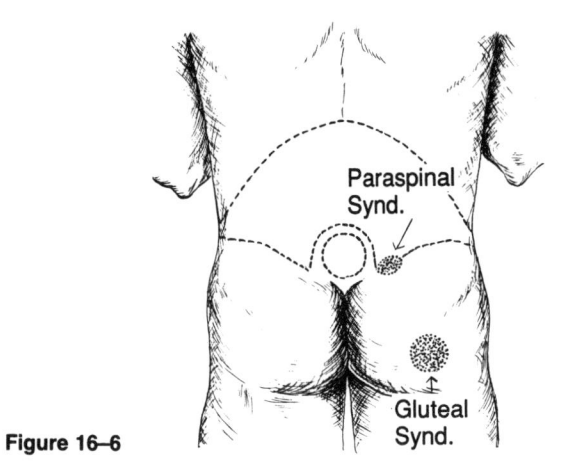

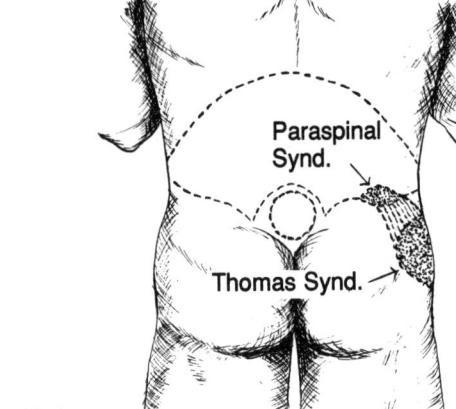

Figure 16-9

Figure 16-10

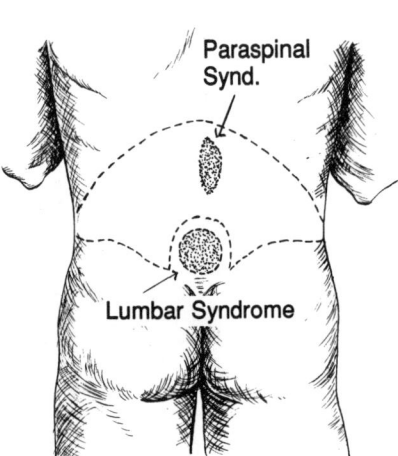

Figure 16-11

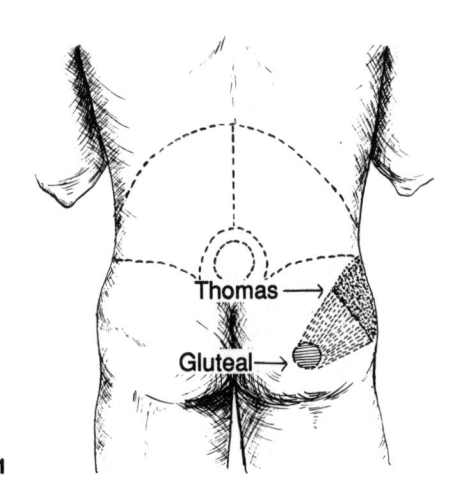

COMPOSITE PAIN SYNDROME 87

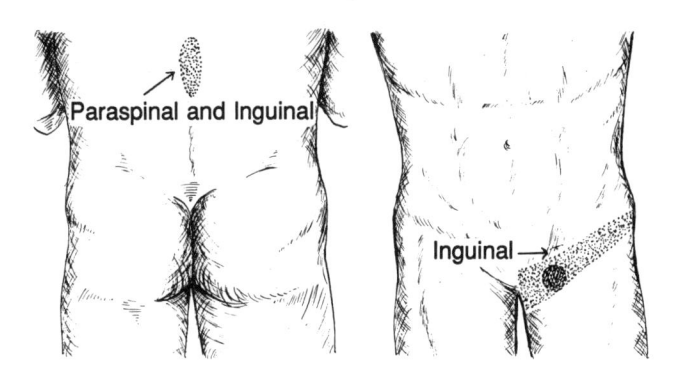

Figure 16–12

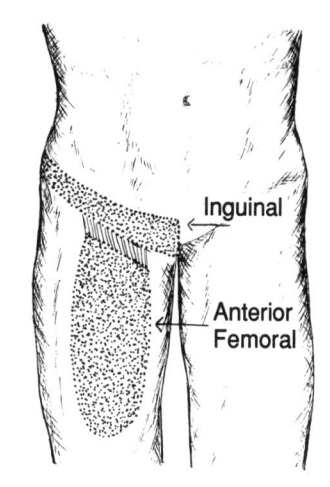

Figure 16–15

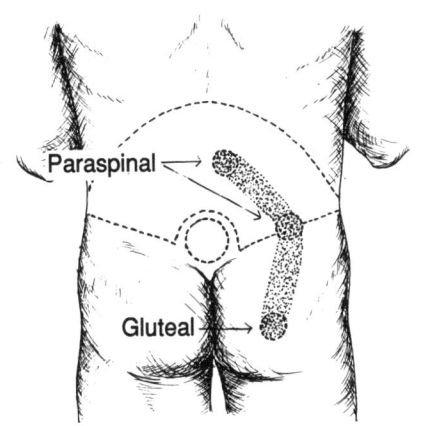

Figure 16–13

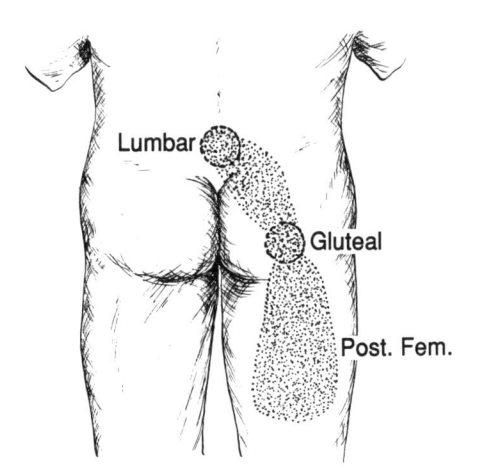

Figure 16–16

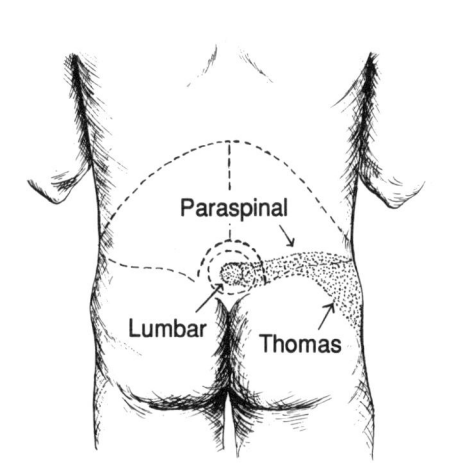

Figure 16–14

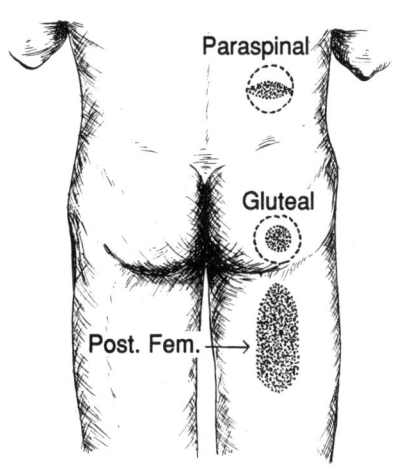

Figure 16–17

Figure 16-18

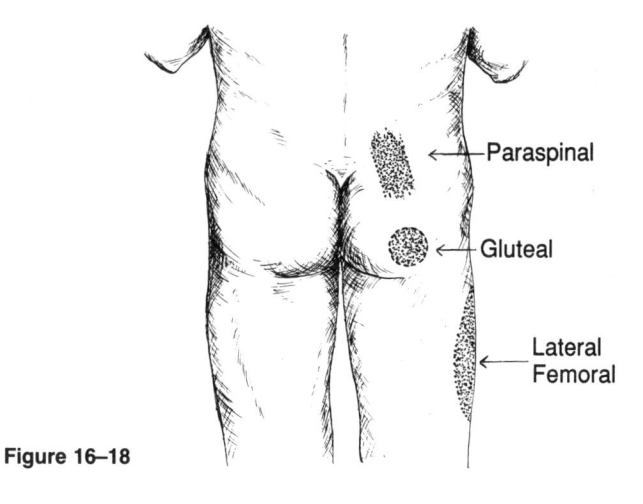

patients have smaller areas of pain found within the pain syndrome area, particularly the paraspinal area.)

Examples of Composite Pain Syndromes

If one considers a torsion injury to the 2nd lumbar vertebra, and envisions the tissue injury that might occur to both the top and bottom of that segment, it is easily understood that pain syndromes neurologically arising from the spinal levels above and below could be present. This includes the paraspinal, inguinal, Thomas, gluteal, anterior, and lateral femoral pain syndromes. Fortunately, this configuration rarely takes place, but the basis for reaction above and below the injured segment is there, and the presence of pain syndromes to those levels should not be surprising.

For example, a patient may have an anterior femoral pain syndrome associated with a paraspinal pain syndrome and found at some point along the iliac crest. The only reactive segment in this case may be the 5th lumbar. A reactive 5th lumbar indicates that the 5th lumbar is a lesion (probably secondary), sending neural impulses upward via the posterior primary rami. The 2nd lumbar neural system receiving these abnormal impulses reacts, causing the anterior femoral pain syndrome. The posterior primary rami at the 12th thoracic or 1st lumbar also receives abnormal impulses, and it reacts in a defensive manner causing muscle contraction. Such muscle contraction may range from mild to severe. (Note: It has been stated previously that the greatest reactive spinal segment must have priority treatment, but it was also indicated that the reactive levels higher in the lumbar plexus should always be considered and evaluated for the entire picture.) There are also other cases in which the higher level, although less reactive, should be the first target for treatment. The 12th thoracic/1st lumbar must be treated initially in order to reduce muscle contraction; the 2nd lumbar causing anterior femoral pain is then treated, followed by treatment to the 5th lumbar if it continues to show a reaction. It is not unusual that reaction from the 5th lumbar segment dissipates following treatment to higher segments.

A second example of anterior femoral pain, with paraspinal pain at some point along the iliac crest, may present a different situation. The spinal segmental examination may indicate a hot or highly reactive 2nd lumbar segment with negative findings below this level. No treatment or consideration should then be given to spinal segments below this level. The anterior femoral pain syndrome arises from the 2nd lumbar level. The 12th thoracic/1st lumbar level, receiving excess neural impulses, reacts in the form of antalgic contraction. This contraction can vary in intensity from case to case and may cause the paraspinal pain syndrome at the iliac crest. Both levels should be treated, although in this case no reaction is noted at the 12th thoracic/1st lumbar level during the segmental examination. Given time, reaction would develop at this upper level.

A third example is presented by the same pain syndromes with a segmental reaction found only at the 12th thoracic/1st lumbar level. This is not uncommon in the presence of an old secondary nonreactive lesion (nonreactive, or mildly reactive to the segmental examination). It appears that the low-grade lesion at the 2nd lumbar sends continuous impulses to the 12th thoracic/1st lumbar level with ultimate reaction from that neural system. This constant reaction may cause pathological changes at the 12th thoracic/1st lumbar level, although it is not the originally injured level. The primary treatment in this case is at the 12th thoracic/1st lumbar level. The 2nd lumbar should be monitored and treated if necessary.

Comprehending the reasons for the presence of the paraspinal pain syndrome facilitates the diagnosis and treatment of low back, pelvic, and leg pain when it is associated with or present within multiple pain syndromes.

Consider an injury to the 5th lumbar spinal level, with the spinal segmental and regional orthopedic examinations positive only at that segment. One could expect local deep muscular reaction, ranging from the 4th lumbar to and including the sacrum, in the form of muscle contraction (posterior primary protective reaction). In many cases, no other neural involvement or segmental reaction is present, particularly during the early period following the injury. When general antalgic contraction is not detected in the form of a paraspinal pain syndrome, or if 12th thoracic/1st lumbar segmental reaction is not detected, the treatment may be confined to the 5th lumbar spinal segment. Should this patient delay treatment, or if treatment has no response, a segmental reaction noted at the 12th thoracic/1st lumbar level will ultimately arise. At that point, treatment is needed at both levels, the upper level first. Further delay in spinal segmental treatment eventually causes pain syndromes from the lumbar plexus.

A severe injury, or a milder, uncorrected injury to the 5th lumbar segment may take the following pattern.

The 5th lumbar is injured, severely or is untreated, or improperly treated: the joint and soft tissue injury creates changes to the vascular and neural systems, which result in the flooding of neural tissues with neural impulses. These abnormal impulses cause the reactions that occur to the posterior and anterior primary rami, and the pain syndromes are the consequence of that irritation. First, local muscle contraction is present; second, general muscle contraction develops, including muscles supplied by both the lumbar and sacral plexus posterior primary rami. These reactions may cause the paraspinal pain syndrome and possibly the gluteal pain syndrome. When the anterior primary rami becomes involved, the inguinal syndrome, Thomas syndrome, anterior femoral, lateral femoral, and posterior femoral pain syndromes may result. In the presence of a 5th lumbar lesion, the posterior femoral pain syndrome is the most common pain area. If the above should occur and both posterior and anterior primary rami are involved, the patient experiences *back pain, groin pain, hip pain, buttock pain, and leg pain*. Every chiropractor who treats low back cases has seen this problem in varying degrees and the diagnosis is frequently a 4th or 5th lumbar disc lesion.

When a case reaches this proportion, almost all the lumbosacral segments show a recording during the spinal segmental examination. These recordings may range from sensitive to highly reactive.

More than one level may fall within the highly reactive range. The reaction at all levels indicates that all portions of the neural system at the lumbosacral plexus are involved in varying degrees. In such cases, the first level to be treated must be the uppermost showing the highest segmental rating, in order to reduce reaction at those levels most responsible for paraspinal antalgic contraction. The reduced contraction then enables the chiropractor to conduct specific segmental manipulation more effectively to the lower segments. Treatment is continued until the segmental reaction is appreciably reduced, and then the lower segments are treated. Resistance to manipulation at the lower levels indicates that muscle contraction is not reduced enough to continue; the physician must revert back to upper-level treatment until this contraction is reduced. The lower level may be treated if considerable caution is exercised.

Many examples could be given. The important factor is the knowledge that both the anterior and posterior primary neural rami are, or may become, involved in low back, pelvic, and leg pain cases. The basic difference between these two rami appears to be related to the protection of the spinal unit. Although the posterior primary rami reaction is expressed by muscle activity in its attempt to protect the spinal unit from further damage at a local level, the anterior primary rami causes pain away from the spine at the areas supplied by the nerve. There is no scientific evidence available that pain resulting from irritation to the anterior primary rami is associated with spinal protective mechanism. We must not, however, eliminate that possibility, although remote. Taking into consideration these factors, and being aware of the individual pain syndromes' characteristics, the physician can conduct the orthopedic and segmental examinations with full knowledge that these procedures reveal basic information regarding complex multiple pain syndromes; such knowledge is an aid in the evaluation of treatment for each individual case.

Chapter 17

Disability Impairment Evaluation for Low Back/Leg Pain

Low back injuries from industrial, auto, and personal accidents are responsible for millions of lost work hours, and untold suffering to those injured.

The financial cost of treatment, diagnosis, hospital care, compensation, court costs, and legal fees amounts to many millions of dollars. These costs are accelerating each year at a staggering rate.[1] Compensation and legal fees resulting from low back injuries are a major portion of these costs. In order to determine the extent of injury and to evaluate the patient's physical impairment, an examination by a physician is necessary. Rules established in 1938 allow any federal court to order a physical examination in liable cases involving injuries.[2]

During the past 30 years, the American Medical Association (AMA) has endeavored to create a guide for rating physical impairment. This necessary guide has included all body systems that, when impaired, can lead to a patient's disability. Each system mentioned, except one, offers symptoms to evaluate and review, various known precise tests that should be utilized, test evaluations that are indicated, examples of individual impaired patients with their physical and laboratory findings, and last, diagnostic procedures with test results that might be expected. The one system devoid of the noted information is "The Extremities, Spine and Pelvis." With its high price tag, the low back injury is a part of this system.[3]

Information on low back/leg pain diagnostic procedures that are necessary to determine a viable impairment evaluation were probably not deliberately deleted from impairment guides. In fact, no structured, reputable examination for low back/leg pain has, to date, been accepted by the healing arts.[4]

It is estimated that only 20 physicians of two million are dedicated to low back pain research.[5]

McBride, author of the reference text *Disability Evaluation* indicates that a scientific procedure must be developed on which a professional opinion can be based.[6]

Currently accepted recommendations for the evaluation of low back/leg pain cases discussed in the third edition of the AMA *Guides to the Evaluation of Permanent Impairment* are presented below.

PROCEDURES PRESENTLY ACCEPTED BY THE AMA GUIDE

1. Measurement of low back flexion and extension, right and left bending, right and left rotation. Impairment rating is determined by increments of 5°, or +/− 10% using a goneometer,[7] or an inclinometer.[8]

2. Reduced or unreduced vertebral dislocation or subluxation. This information regarding the subluxation is found in the second edition of the *Guides*, in the section entitled "The Spine," page 46. It is, however, deleted from that section in the third edition and placed under "Upper Extremities," where the term *vertebra* is deleted. It was not listed under lower extremities (see the third edition, page 45). Although it is true that a subluxation can be produced to upper extremity joints, it is not unique to that area. All joints, including the lower extremity and spinal joints, are subject to subluxation. The placement in this area may well have been an error.

   Information for the third edition states that the small, inaccessible spinal joints are not easily observed, nor easily measured externally, and that the measurement of spinal movement can be highly inaccurate when using the goniometer. The inclinometer is now recommended by the AMA for measuring gross spinal motion. (Dislocation and reduced dislocation are mentioned

and assigned values in the *Guides,* third edition, page 73, Table 49.)
3. Several named conditions are rated on an individual basis and therefore not considered in this book (gross pathology).
4. Individual peripheral spinal nerves and muscles supplied by those nerves are shown, arising from the 12th thoracic to the 4th sacral spinal levels. An analysis for impairment evaluation is made for each nerve named and for the lumbosacral plexus. The spinal nerves listed are from the anterior primary rami, but small portions of the dorsal rami of the 12th thoracic are shown, and the body area from the 1st, 2nd, and 3rd sacral are shown. Various tables are also shown that could aid the physician in the rating procedure.

As each point previously listed is discussed, certain facts must be considered. Low back injuries may be superimposed upon constitutional diseases of bone, birth defects, and other pathologies existing at the time of injury.[9] Although gross pathologies do not ordinarily cause a diagnostic problem, injuries superimposed upon many of these pathologies may invalidate any impairment ratings if the determination is based only upon motion studies.

If these conditions are compensable when associated with a low back injury, it might be of greater value to the adjudicator to rate the existing gross pathology separately from the low back injury. This would not prevent the doctor from showing the reactive relationships between the two conditions; in fact, it might provide a clearer or more accurate picture of each. The court then has the option of evaluating the patient's disability on either a separate or a combined basis. This concept is not entirely new. In its application, however, it is necessary to be able to separate the accidental spinal joint dysfunction and pathology from gross spinal changes of constitutional diseases or previous injury. This cannot be done by considering only the ability of the body to move within certain ranges using motion studies, but must be determined by the reaction of the individual joint.

The objective in rating a disability is to diagnose and record the structural changes that occur within the body that reduce established physical abilities.[10] This goal in low back/leg pain syndromes is difficult at best, and every effort should be made to control and upgrade procedures to enable the doctor to attain this objective with as little variance as possible.

Motion studies are highly effective for the determination of gross spinal pathological changes that cause restriction in tested movements. Many joint changes can occur that do not affect motion ranges in an office setting. Hypermobile joints, facet subluxation, torsion injuries[11] and even isolated pathological changes may not restrict motion during routine physical testing. Offering the range of motion as a major means of determining physical impairment, the present system does not take into account all forms of low back injuries or functional impairment that might exist. The patient with a functionally impaired spinal joint who is able to move within a near normal range for the examination may be rated normal using this guide, and yet could not work more than a few minutes without severe pain.

(On page 72 of the *Guides,* third edition, it is stated that future editions will include task performance capabilities. This would certainly be of great assistance in cases of functional impairment, rather than from reduced regional motion on a limited basis. In the interval, however, these cases must be evaluated as best as possible.

The second procedure for impairment evaluation, titled "Vertebral—Dislocation or Subluxation" is found in the *Guides,* second edition. Because a spinal dislocation would rarely if ever be seen in a private office, it may not be necessary to discuss it in this book, but because it is a major cause of low back/leg pain, it must be determined for impairment factors.

Serious injury can occur to spinal joints. The latest research indicates that disc lesions, lateral entrapment, and traumatic arthritis are a sequel to the unreduced subluxation.[12] Torsion injury also causes a stretch to nerve roots and instability associated with joint and disc damage.[13] Reports showing spinal joint injury and dysfunction are increasing at a rapid rate; these reports are not confined to the United States.[14]

An accepted spinal segmental examination would aid in the differential diagnosis of spinal joint pathology, and it would be an effective adjunct to present impairment evaluation procedures.

The last procedure, spinal nerve impairment, has been simplified as much as possible, using the available knowledge. Individual nerves have been rated and nerve roots are shown with their locations in the plexus and their spinal levels of origin. The muscles innervated by these nerves are visualized and several tables are drawn, providing additional specific information.

Regardless of this analysis of the complex neural system, low back/leg pain cases continue to remain one of the major problems in differential diagnosis, and this difficulty is reflected in the physical impairment ratings.

In his book, McBride seems to sum up the problems with these words, "The situation cannot be remedied except by the development of some practicable, scientific procedure on which a professional opinion can be based."[10]

The purpose of this chapter is not to create a new, untested impairment evaluation system, but rather to utilize the present system in the most efficient manner possible for all low back/leg pain cases. With this goal, the anatomical structures that can be affected are reviewed below.

Anatomical Structures

The anatomical structures most frequently subject to injury or reaction from the injury to the low back include the following.

1. Any of the spinal joints found from the 10th thoracic to the 5th lumbar spinal level, including a total of 16 posterior arthrodial joints. These joints are subject to the same type of changes that occur to other body joints: degeneration, arthritis, and joint destruction.
2. The neural posterior primary rami found at these same spinal levels, including their interlinking nerve systems.
3. The recurrent sinuvertebral nerve, a branch from the posterior primary rami, at the same spinal level.
4. The anterior primary rami found at each spinal level and the pain syndrome areas resulting from their injury.
5. Low back muscles associated with spinal motion that produce spinal splinting as a protective mechanism.
6. The disc, subject to immediate injury or delayed changes leading to disc degeneration.
7. The vascular system, which may be adversely affected and contribute to further neural injury.
8. Other soft tissue such as ligaments, periosteum, and fascia, which may become involved in low back injuries, with ultimate fibrotic changes.

Determination of Pain Syndromes

The first step is to obtain an accurate location of the pain from the patient, following a very specific procedure.[15]

The procedure is to obtain an accurate location of pain from the patient before any other form of examination is attempted. The chiropractor asks the patient to indicate the area of pain and outline this area as closely as possible. This should begin at the low back region, progress to the pelvis, and conclude with the leg region. These pain areas are to be sketched or shaded on a body drawing, using both front and back views. Lateral body drawings give additional perspective.

A manual examination determines the area of pain. Without this predetermination of actual pain areas suffered by the patient, the doctor is led beyond those pain boundaries and is frequently misled. An inaccurate diagnosis is then the ultimate result.

When the pain syndrome is identified, it must be charted on a body drawing designed for that purpose, to establish a permanent record. This drawing is a constant reminder of the area of pain suffered by the patient. It is a highly effective means of communication between other physicians and third parties.

It cannot then be distorted or misinterpreted by anyone. There are eight major pain syndromes found in low back/leg pain cases. A patient with a low back injury may suffer from one, two, or multiple pain syndromes. Each one should be determined individually, just as they were previously mentioned and charted individually.[15]

Physical Examination

Two very specific examination procedures should be conducted in every low back/leg pain case.

1. The regional orthopedic examination, to determine the extent of injury to the various low back and leg tissues. (The examination is shown in Chapter 6.)
2. Segmental spinal examination, to determine the integrity of each spinal joint and its related structures. (The segmental spinal examination is shown in Chapter 7).

All findings, both negative and positive, should be recorded no matter how seemingly insignificant.

Other Examination Procedures

Anterior–posterior and lateral spinal pilot x-rays are necessary and should be the minimum required, but they show only gross pathology when it is present. The field of view from the 10th thoracic to the sacrum is essential to viewing the entire low back region. Lateral flexion studies, obliques, and spot films can be left to the discretion of the chiropractor, but lateral flexion studies will frequently show variations in the ability of motor units to function and should be taken if there is any question as to the cause of pain.

Diagnostic ultrasound, MRI, and CAT scans of the spine may be used in some cases. If these diagnostic procedures are considered, they should follow the dictates of the spinal segmental examination and nerve root level of the pain syndrome as shown. Scans taken at other levels often show false-positive readings of tissue areas not involved in the pain syndrome.[16] At present, thermograms do not show the actual pain area suffered by the patient, and are, therefore, of little value for chronic low back/leg pain syndromes. The EMG will, however, show the paraspinal muscle contraction utilized by the body as a defense mechanism. This contraction is caused by a reaction from the posterior primary rami and is highly effective in visualizing the presence of the objective antalgic contraction.[17]

The author's statistical research has shown that low back spinal injuries affect patients in the following percentages.

1. Low back pain only	54%
2. Nerve root or radiating pain only	22%
3. Both combined	24%

Depending upon the severity of the injury, either of these pain situations can result in loss of spinal motion, functional stability, or both. Because the causes of loss in gross spinal motion are usually quite evident, they will not be discussed here. This leaves functional spinal impairment and minimal spinal motion loss as our targets.

To avoid confusion, the three body regions for low back, pelvic, and leg pain are discussed separately (see Chapter 1, Fig. 1–1).

1. Low back region
2. Pelvic region
3. Leg region

The first consideration is pain found in the low back region resulting from a spinal injury.

In order to give a proper impairment evaluation for the low back region, the pain found in that region must be understood.

There appears to be a natural division separating three pain areas: Segmental examination of more than 7000 spinal vertebrae has shown that the 3rd lumbar vertebral motor unit is less frequently injured and is seldom reactive even when spinal x-rays indicate pathology is present. This phenomenon enables the chiropractor to separate or distinguish injuries above or below this apparent barrier and to determine if both areas are involved.

1. Unless severe, injuries below the 3rd lumbar, to the 4th or 5th lumbar motor units confine the pain syndrome to a close circle over the lumbosacral joint. Examination procedures described confirm this area. Severe injury at this level demands protective antalgic muscle contraction. Neural impulses activate the nervous system at the 9th, 10th, 11th, and 12th thoracic levels, and 1st lumbar nerve to create spinal splinting. The spinal segments 11th, and 12th thoracic, and 1st lumbar are reactive to probing. The 12th thoracic is usually extremely painful.

   When the 4th or 5th lumbar units are not involved, the examination shows negative findings at the lumbosacral joint. Pain in the supraspinal ligament on probing, or during the straight leg raising (SLR) test may be caused by injury to any spinal segments found in the low back region. This pain syndrome must be differentiated from the lumbar syndrome caused by 4th or 5th lumbar injury. From an impairment evaluation standpoint, however, the persistence of this pain area still constitutes a lumbar pain syndrome.

2. Injuries above the 3rd lumbar level, especially to the 11th and 12th thoracic, and 1st lumbar, cause pain from 1½ to 2 inches lateral to the center line of the lumbosacral joint, extending along the iliac crest, both above and below it. These pain areas are diagnostic for injuries or reaction from the lumbar plexus posterior primary rami. Examination of paraspinal muscles show contraction, and pain will overlay these muscles at some point.

3. The third pain area is also found along the iliac crest, above and slightly below it, involving the quadratus lumborum. This muscle response may range from tense to a severe contraction. Pain along its attachment and upon probing indicates its involvement in the pain syndrome. Body posture is affected in severe cases and may be diagnostic for quadratus lumborum contraction. This muscle is supplied by the anterior primary rami from the 1st lumbar spinal unit. The 12th thoracic nerve seems to be intimately associated with this pain syndrome, as it is always reactive to probing when the 1st lumbar is involved.

Severe injury to the 5th lumbar joint may demand antalgic muscle contraction for protection of the joint.[18] When this occurs, spinal nerves supplying muscles of motion are activated. The neural spinal levels are the 9th, 10th, 11th, and 12th thoracic, and the 1st lumbar. These nerves and their associated spinal joints may become involved in the total injury complex.

Chronic loss of motion may produce joint injury with biochemical and histological changes[19] at these levels, although these changes are not the focus of the original injury. When this action results from injury, although it is a secondary reaction, it is a part of the total injury, and so subject to impairment rating. The regional and segmental examination confirms this state. Each joint injured from the reaction must be rated accordingly.

Should the anterior primary rami become involved from injury to either the principal or secondary area, the existence of the pain syndrome supplied neurologically from that area must be present in order to rate it.

The two pain syndromes, the paraspinal and lumbar syndromes, found in the low back region have just been described showing their relationship to low back injuries.

1. Paraspinal syndrome
2. Lumbar syndrome

Three pain syndromes are found in the pelvic region.

1. Inguinal syndrome
2. Gluteal syndrome
3. Thomas syndrome

These pain syndromes indicate injury to or tissue reaction changes from the anterior primary rami.

1. The inguinal pain syndrome found on the anterior side of the pelvic region is caused by spinal motor unit injury, and is a part of low back/leg pain syndromes.

    Two pain areas are found in this syndrome. One or both may be present due to spinal injury. Impairment ratings may have to be considered for both areas.

2. The gluteal pain syndrome found in the pelvic region is also caused by spinal joint injury. It occurs in 3% of all single pain syndrome cases.

    An impairment rating required for this syndrome should rate its posterior primary rami involvement on the same basis as an anterior primary rami injury. It is commonly found in conjunction with other pain syndromes; when present as a composite injury it still should be rated separately.

3. The Thomas syndrome is also found in two parts and is caused by spinal joint injury. Either or both pain areas may be present and may have to be rated separately.

Three pain syndromes are found in the leg region. Their nerve supply is also from the anterior primary nerve division.

1. Anterior femoral pain syndrome
2. Lateral femoral pain syndrome
3. Posterior femoral pain syndrome

1. The nerve supply for the anterior femoral pain syndromes arises from the lumbar plexus.
2. The nerve supply for the lateral femoral pain syndrome arises from the lumbar plexus.
3. The sciatic nerve arises from the sacral plexus, and may cause pain to the posterior femoral syndrome area.

    The posterior femoral nerve arises from the sacral plexus via metamerism and causes pain to the posterior femoral syndrome area.

Segregating the lumbar and sacral plexuses from one another enables the chiropractor to utilize them independently or collectively in impairment rating values. This is one more means of clearing the air so that third parties can have a better understanding of the tissues injured or impaired.

DISCUSSION RELATED TO IMPAIRMENT RATING

The most complex cases confronting the chiropractor when considering an impairment evaluation are those no longer having pain in areas of the body supplied by the anterior primary rami, or those in which anterior rami involvement was never present. Any case with continued pain and muscle weakness to this neural system can easily be rated using tables found in the third edition of the *Guides*, under single or combined nerve or nerve groups. The greatest problem in these cases is the explanation as to why continued symptoms exist when gross pathology is not present. The reader should now be able to discuss disrelation lesions and the manner in which their reduced load limits cause symptoms, and also able to explain the sequel to these lesions. The determination of a rating for those impaired spinal joints that are less than gross lesions is most difficult because the text of the *Guides* has not made provisions for this type of lesion.

The neural system closely associated with spinal joint pathology and joint reaction is the posterior primary rami, which controls the muscles of motion, its response in the form of antalgic contraction of deep spinal muscles, and the reduced joint load limit resulting from permanent joint and surrounding soft-tissue damage. A large percentage of this type of case cannot be accurately rated using regional motion as a method of measurement, unless the patient is tested during a period of increased reaction. This is not recommended by the *Guides*.

In the *Guides* (ref. 3, page 71), it is stated that acute antalgic spasm is a phenomenon caused by a recent increase in the load limit, causing an overload, and that this state is a contraindication to the assessment of impairment, at that point in time. This is an acceptable statement, and the author agrees that a patient should not be evaluated during an acute stage of antalgic spasm. When the acute spasm is reduced, it changes only the muscle response to the joint injury, but does not change the reduced joint load limit or the patient's reduced functional ability. The acute antalgic contraction returns each and every time the patient exceeds that load limit, thus defining him or her as impaired. When a patient's condition becomes static and stabilized following all rehabilitative treatment, he or she is then ready for evaluation. It is at this point that joint reaction can be determined by the segmental examination, and the presence of chronic or permanent antalgic pathological contraction can be noted.

An impairment evaluation for low back injuries is considered in the following steps.

1. A permanent impairment rating for spinal injuries that does not show gross pathology should rarely be considered less than 1 year from the date of injury. This usually allows ample time for treatment during the acute stage, and a period of tissue repair and rehabilitation. Joints, nerves, and soft tissue that are permanently damaged can then be assessed with reasonable confidence.

    If the chiropractor is sure that the presence of gross pathology is caused by the injury related to the impairment rating required and that the condition is static at an earlier date than 1 year, impairment rating may then be assigned, if requested.
2. Only those joints injured and reactive from the injury, either primary or secondary, are considered for rating. An example is a 5th lumbar motor unit injury: antalgic reaction involves the 12th thoracic unit. Segmental examination indicates that these two units are part of the injured area. X-rays confirm arthritis at the 3rd lumbar joint during the initial spinal examination. The segmental examination is negative at that level and remains negative during the acute stage. Later, when an impairment rating is necessary, the 3rd lumbar joint must not be rated as part of the original injury.
3. The nervous system is rather complex, but if certain guidelines are followed, rating can be accomplished relatively easily.

    Two major divisions of the nervous system may become reactive due to joint injury. Each side of the body is supplied neurologically by anterior and posterior primary divisions of the spinal nerves. Either or both may become involved with spinal joint injury. These nerve rami are found at each spinal segmental level of the low back and, when reactive due to injury, produce pain that is found within known pain syndrome areas. Each neural system and each side of the body should be considered and rated separately.

The determination of ranges of gross spinal motion will not be discussed in this chapter as it is well covered in the third edition of the *Guides*.

It should be mentioned that in the absence of gross pathology, some physicians minimize reduced ranges of motion. I have read many reports of reduced motion, some as much as 35%, with the physician's summation stating that the patient was able to return to full activity.

The principal concern in this chapter is the impairment evaluation of nongross lesions: lesions that produce permanent, persistent antalgic contraction causing restricted joint motion and reduced joint function. Individual joints, or even two or three restricted joints within a spinal region, may cause little regional limited motion and in some cases no perceptible limited motion during an examination or regional motion study. The load limit for a permanently damaged joint is reduced in varying degrees depending upon the tissues injured. If the patient does not exceed the permanently decreased load limit of the joint, he or she may be relatively free of pain, but this does not indicate that the joint problem is normal, whether of pathological or functional origin. This remains true although a regional motion study may be negative. Such a finding indicates that regional motion examinations as now used are not a proper evaluation procedure for permanently injured joint lesions with functional impairment.

The following information in the evaluation of impairment of a reactive spinal lesion must be considered.

- As previously mentioned, the third edition of the *Guides* (page 45) rates persistent joint subluxation in upper extremity joints as mild, completely reduced; moderate, partially reduced; and severe, cannot be reduced. Because a subluxation may affect all joints of the body, particularly spinal joints, this guide can be used as a further aid in evaluating the joint. When joints continue to be reactive to 4 to 6 pounds pressure during the segmental examination at the time an impairment rating is recommended, the reaction is rated as mild, painful, sharp, or highly reactive. An evaluation arrived at in this manner does not depend upon either the fixation, or instability of the joint, but rather on its pathological reaction to minor movements produced by the segmental examination procedure.
- Although a mild spinal segmental reaction is rarely considered for an impairment rating, it is not impossible. The evaluation of the joint would probably look like this:

Persistent Joint Subluxation		Segmental Rating	% IMP.
Mild =	Completely reduced	Pain	20
Moderate =	Cannot be permanently reduced	Sharp	40
Severe =	Cannot be permanently reduced	Highly reactive	60

Although the use of this chart does not indicate differences in the completed impairment rating figures, and the impairment percentage as shown cannot be used by following the AMA guidelines for spinal lesions, it offers a basis for diagnostic findings by showing that a subluxation can vary in its impairment. Thus, the physician is allowed some latitude in the final impairment evaluation for reactive spinal segments.

Because the third edition of the *Guides* does not show that nongross lesions causes functional impairment, when rated separately, the physician must use evaluation tables that are less than ideal for these lesions. Hence, it is advisable to refer to Table 49, page 73 and Table 50, page 79. Table 49 presents impairments due to specific joint pathology, and Table 50 is used for those joints that are ankylosed (complete absence of motion or restrictions that prevent the spinal segment from returning to a normal neutral or resting position). Tables 11a and 11b can also be used to evaluate the strength of the region. As discussed before, however, regional evaluation differs from segmental evaluation, and an attempt to use this table may not be satisfactory in many spinal joint cases.

Spinal lesions that involve only the posterior primary rami produce pain in the low back region. This is an area in low back cases ranging from the 10th thoracic to and including the sacrum and its surrounding soft-tissue area. Areas of pain can extend along the iliac crest, both above and below the crest. In some cases, the gluteal pain will be present.

Rating an Impaired Spinal Joint

When a spinal segmental examination generates persistent reactivity in a joint or spinal joints following a reasonable period of treatment and rehabilitation, and has a reduced load limit as evidenced by the patient's lessened ability to perform normal activities that could have been performed previously, an impairment rating should be assigned.

The chiropractor must indicate the reactive spinal segment or segments, the posterior primary nerve from that level, and the muscle or muscle group that is chronically contracted and subject to pain. Muscle groups such as the rotatores, multifidus, longissimus thoracis, interspinales etc., are identified. When a reasonable evaluation of individual muscle groups cannot be differentiated, the sacrospinalis can be listed.

There are two areas in Table 49 (*Guides*, page 73) that can be used in the rating of spinal lesions.

1. Section C, #1, denotes "reduced dislocation of one vertebra." (A subluxation and a dislocation rank equally in this consideration, page 45, "Persistent Joint Subluxation and Dislocation.") Furthermore, the second edition, page 45, "Vertebrae—Dislocation or Subluxation," can be used as a precedent.
2. Section B, #2, unoperated, soft tissue lesions. This shows a rating of 5% of the whole person for one vertebra. Number one will probably be used in most cases.

Section C, #2, is a patient with limited motion and could be rated under standard motion ranges.

Lumbar vertebra: Section C, #1

One lumbar vertebra: 6% impairment of whole person
If two or more vertebrae require an impairment rating, use the AMA Combined Values Chart in the third edition, pages 246 and 247

Thoracic vertebrae: Section C, #1

> One thoracic vertebra: 3% impairment of whole person
> If two or more vertebrae require an impairment rating, use the AMA Combined Values Chart in the third edition, on pages 246 and 247

Table 50 on page 79 can be used to determine impairment by x-ray. This table should be used only when motion study x-rays such as flexion, extension, and lateral flexion films are taken and the motion measured for each segment, showing a definite reduction of joint motion. The basic position of the vertebra above and below can easily be determined as favorable or unfavorable.

(Note that the 12th thoracic and 1st lumbar are rated together and are commonly found injured or reactive in a combined state; also note at the bottom of the chart, impairment of several segments with ankylosis (reduced motion) are indicated and rated as a group.)

The ratings as previously shown are only for spinal joint impairment and do not include all neural injury to the anterior primary rami or posterior primary rami. Nerve injury caused by joint pathology must be rated separately.

Rating an Impaired Posterior Primary Rami

Following joint impairment, the posterior primary rami must be considered. (*Guides,* page 66, Fig. 79 shows both rami). (Note that the terms, dorsal rami and posterior rami, as well as anterior rami and ventral rami are frequently used interchangeably.)

1. If only those muscles surrounding the reactive spinal segment are reactive, painful, or contracted, they should be considered part of the joint segmental impairment.
2. Muscles that extend away from the joint, one attachment to a part of the body other than the spine, or a reactive muscle that is not a part of the joint, must be considered separately and rated; then its rating is combined with the joint rating, using the combined value chart at the end of the *Guides,* third edition.
3. The most common muscle groups that fall in this category requiring an impairment rating are the longissimus and the gluteus. Either constant or intermittent chronic pain in these groups, with associated spinal joint injury, require their separate rating.

The areas of pain are most commonly found at the iliac crest, above or below and at the sacral attachment.

The *Guides* text has not named the above muscle groups, but their rating should be no less than soft-tissue lesions as listed in Table 49, #2B.

> Longissimus muscles—impairment loss, 5% whole body
> Gluteal muscles—impairment loss, 5% whole body
> Use combined values chart at the end of the book combining muscle lesion with joint lesion

The two following muscle groups are listed separately because their involvement usually causes motion impairment in their own right, and each is caused by spinal joint subluxation/disrelation lesions.

1. The quadratus lumborum, a muscle of the low back region, is supplied by the anterior primary nerve division. Its function is important in spinal motion and should be rated equally with other anterior primary rami. (Refer to schematic on quadratus lumborum muscle, Chapter 5, Fig. 5–3.)

> RATE: 5% of the whole body

2. The cluneal nerves, gluteal pain syndrome, part of the lumbar posterior primary division, causes a pain syndrome in the pelvic region and is also affected by body motion. A member of the posterior primary rami, this nerve group must be rated similarly to anterior primary rami nerves that cause pain away from the low back region.

> RATE: 5% of the whole body

Ratings for these two groups must be combined with the joint lesion as noted in the previous groups.

The nerve divisions discussed include the paraspinal, lumbar, and gluteal pain syndromes.

Rating an Impaired Anterior Primary Rami

The following pain syndromes are supplied by the

anterior primary nerve division. (Refer to schematic on anterior primary rami, Chapter 16, Fig. 16–1.)

Table 47, page 70, third edition of the *Guides* should be used as a reference guide.

The Thomas and inguinal pain syndromes are unique in that they are both neurologically supplied by the same nerve group and the same spinal level. Each syndrome also has two pain areas. Each area appears to represent nerve irritation from a different nerve, as both areas are not always present.

The nerve group is the 12th thoracic/1st lumbar with its combined nerves, the iliohypogastric and ilioinguinal. The 12th thoracic motor unit is involved in 86.5% of all cases in these two syndromes. The schematic shows the most common nerves associated with these pain areas. For an impairment evaluation to specifically identify each nerve places an unnecessary burden on the physician and may also be controversial.

This nerve group rates the percentage of loss of function and must be converted to the impairment of the whole body by using Table 42, page 65 in the third edition of the *Guides*.

The Thomas and inguinal pain syndromes are rated in the following manner:

```
Rate:  One pain area—5% loss of function
       Two pain areas—8% loss of function
```

This method of rating would bypass all deviations that might occur to the neural linkage described.

The following pain syndromes are found in the leg region.

A. Anterior femoral
B. Lateral femoral
C. Posterior femoral

A. The anterior femoral syndrome area is supplied from the femoral nerve, spinal levels 2nd, 3rd, and 4th lumbar segments. Injury to the lumbar plexus or sacral plexus may cause this pain syndrome. Because, however, the 4th lumbar joints are not frequently reactive in these pain cases, it would appear that the most responsible level falls within the lumbar plexus.

(It is interesting to note that during research in every case with anterior femoral pain, the 12th thoracic motor unit was injured or reactive. Hence, the author believes that antalgic contraction of the spinal levels involved may be one cause of anterior femoral pain.)

Not shown on the schematics of the anterior femoral pain syndrome is the infrequent pain extension of this syndrome. The knee or the distribution of the saphenous nerve to the great toe may be affected.[20] If this configuration is present when an impairment evaluation is needed, the condition is more severe.

```
Rate:  Anterior femoral syndrome — 5% loss of
                                   function
       Knee and/or saphenous — 3% loss of
                                function
```

B. The lateral femoral syndrome is supplied by the lateral femoral cutaneous nerve arising from the 2nd and 3rd spinal lumbar levels. The 12th thoracic motor unit is reactive in 92% of these cases. Joint injury, antalgic contractions, or both due to dorsolumbar injury appear to be the primary cause of this syndrome.

There is no evidence that this syndrome, properly evaluated, is subject to permanent injury on a greater basis than the anterior femoral syndrome.

Although it is rated at 10% in the *Guides'* third edition (page 70, Table 47), it would be more realistically rated at 5%. (Refer to Chapter 14, Lateral Femoral Syndrome.)

When knee or lower leg minor pain syndromes are associated, one rates at an additional 3%. (Note the rating of the anterior femoral syndrome.)

```
Rate:  Lateral femoral syndrome — 5% loss of
                                  function
       Knee, etc. —3% loss of function
```

C. The posterior femoral syndrome arises from the posterior femoral cutaneous nerve via metamerism from the 5th lumbar spinal level. This syndrome is complex, involving the 5th lumbar spinal motor unit along with the 12th thoracic segment, which is reactive in 52% of the cases. This indicates that injury activates paraspinal contraction of low back muscles for protection in many cases.

Permanent impairment of this nerve constitutes a greater threat to the patient and is rated higher. When its communicating nerve, the sural, is associated as a pain syndrome, the impairment is even greater.[21]

> Rate: Posterior femoral nerve —10% loss of function
> Sural nerve —5% loss of function

The great sciatic nerve is also responsible for pain to the back of the leg, posterior femoral pain syndrome area, and must be rated for impairment when present. The rating for this nerve is shown in Table 47, page 70, the third edition of the *Guides*. The rating there is easily understood, and it is not necessary to repeat it in this text.

> **(When a neurological rating is given, it is necessary to indicate the area of pain suffered by the patient, the nerve supply to that area of pain, the spinal level or levels from which the nerve supply arises, and some information as to the type of impairment caused by the pain syndrome.**
> By providing this information, the chiropractor complies with the required guidelines as shown on page 66, third edition of the *AMA Guides to the Evaluation of Permanent Impairment*.

REFERENCES

1. Cox JM: *Low Back Pain,* 4th ed. Baltimore, Williams & Wilkins, 1985;p.1
2. McBride ED: *Disability Evaluation,* 6th ed. Philadelphia, Lippincott, 1963;p.15
3. American Medical Association: *Guides to the Evaluation of Permanent Impairment,* 3rd ed. Chicago, American Medical Association, 1988;p.1
4. American Medical Association: *Guides to the Evaluation of Permanent Impairment,* 3rd ed. Chicago, American Medical Association, 1988;p.215
5. Cox JM: *Low Back Pain,* 4th ed. Baltimore, Williams & Wilkins, 1985;p.4
6. McBride ED: *Disability Evaluation,* 6th ed. Philadelphia, Lippincott, 1963;p.15
7. American Medical Association: *Guides to the Evaluation of Permanent Impairment,* 3rd ed. Chicago, American Medical Association, 1988;p.53
8. American Medical Association: *Guides to the Evaluation of Permanent Impairment,* 3rd ed. Chicago, American Medical Association, 1988;p.53
9. American Medical Association: *Guides to the Evaluation of Permanent Impairment,* 3rd ed. Chicago, American Medical Association, 1988;p.486
10. McBride ED: *Disability Evaluation,* 6th ed. Philadelphia, Lippincott, 1963;p.1
11. McBride ED: *Disability Evaluation,* 6th ed. Philadelphia, Lipponcott, 1963;p.1
12. Farfan HF: The use of mechanical etiology to determine the efficacy of active intervention in single joint lumbar intervertebral joint problems. *Spine* 10(4):350, 1985
13. Farfan HF: The use of mechanical etiology to determine the efficacy of active intervention in single joint lumbar intervertebral joint problems. *Spine* 10(4):350, 1985
14. Farfan HF: The use of mechanical etiology to determine the efficacy of active intervention in single joint lumbar intervertebral joint problems. *Spine* 10(4):350, 1985
15. Mierau DR, Cassidy JD, Hamin T: Sacroiliac joint dysfunction and low back pain in school-aged children. *JMPT* 7(2):81, 1984
16. Thomas J: Classification of low back/leg pain syndromes, Part 2. *FCA Journal* November-December: 39, 1985
17. Pevester RG, Teplic JG, Haskin ME: Computed tomography of lumbosacral conjoined nerve root anomalies. *Spine* 10(4):331, 1985
18. Good AB: Spinal joint blocking. *JMPT* 8(1):1, 1985
19. Dishman R: Review of the literature supporting a scientific basis for the chiropractic subluxation complex. *JMPT* 8(3):163, 1985
20. Gray H: *Gray's Anatomy,* 30th ed. Philadelphia, Lea & Febiger, 1984;p.989
21. Gray H: *Gray's Anatomy,* 30th ed. Philadelphia, Lea & Febiger, 1984;p.998

Chapter 18

Evaluation of Treatment for Low Back/Leg Pain

The treatment for low back/leg pain at present includes almost every method available to the doctor. This includes specific and nonspecific manipulation, all forms of physiotherapy including ultrasound, diathermy, sine wave, traction, rollers, tens, massage, etc. Exercise is often prescribed in active or passive forms by some doctors, whereas others recommend intermittent to total bed rest. All types of pain medication including both nonprescription and prescription drugs are used. Medical practitioners may also recommend nonpain medication that has desirable physiological reactions. Occasionally, patients are sent to specialized physicians or counselors because it is felt that emotional problems are the basis for their low back/leg pain problem. The ultimate treatment for low back/leg pain is surgical intervention. This may range from spinal joint injections to major surgery. This method of treatment, however, should not be used until it is certain that conservative treatment in the form of specific spinal joint manipulation is not efficient.

The probability is that in certain individual cases any of the forms of treatment mentioned above may be, or may appear to be, adequate. The point is that treatment should be determined in accordance with the diagnosis and given with reasonable assurance that it is correct and effective. The current variety of treatment is, however, utilized because of the lack of basic knowledge related to the primary cause of low back/leg pain and its relationship to the specific areas of that pain. When the diagnostic and examination procedures outlined in this manual are followed correctly and conducted consistently for every case of low back, pelvic, and leg pain, the information will develop into a database that will enhance the ability to evaluate each case for the treatment that is best for the individual situation. As this database is further developed, it can be expanded to include all the various forms of treatment. When added to the basic database, the data from each treatment form will then give all physicians an opportunity to determine its value. In time, treatment of little or no value will be discontinued.

The spinal lesion, which is the major cause of the low back, pelvic, and leg pain that has been discussed in this manual, is a generic lesion less than a dislocation. It may not be possible at this time to totally identify each specific tissue injured in any given case, or the precise scientific manner in which injured tissues interact with one another, there are, nevertheless, both subjective and objective signs that when properly determined enable the chiropractor to arrive at the diagnosis of this generic lesion, and to plan the appropriate type of treatment.

When pain is caused by a spinal joint contusion, it indicates that local tissue reaction is sufficient to cause irritation or direct injury to members of the nervous system. This neural involvement appears to be located at or proximate to the spinal segmental foramen. The joint and surrounding soft tissue damage does not differ greatly from similar contusions found at other joints. Spinal joints, however, do have the disc and nerve roots that differentiate this joint from others, and swelling caused by increased tissue flooding is confined within this interforamenal space. Damage to the vascular supply also reduces the ability for the normal interchange related to nutrition, blood chemistry, elimination of toxins, etc. When these soft-tissue reactions occur, and indirect pressure, chemical changes or both involve the nerve root, pain is the sequel. In some cases, the injury is great enough to cause direct nerve pressure by injury to the spinal disc, with protrusion or fragmentation of that disc. Statistics have, however, shown that the latter is found in a very small percentage of these cases.

When treatment for the subluxation/disrelation

spinal lesion is considered, it must first be classified as a primary or secondary lesion. This classification must be based upon the patient history, orthopedic and spinal segmental examinations, and x-ray findings. In many cases, this will be a first-time spinal injury, the patient seeking medical treatment shortly following an accident. The treatment for an acute reaction from a primary spinal joint injury may differ from an acute reaction resulting from injury to a secondary spinal lesion. The immediate reduction of the primary subluxation/disrelation lesion is of vital importance, and specific manipulation to that joint to accomplish this should be done as soon as possible.

This manual is not written for the purpose of describing the techniques related to treatment, but because manipulation has been shown to be highly effective for low back, pelvic, and leg pain syndromes, it is appropriate to discuss this method of treatment in a little more detail.

> **WARNING**
> Spinal manipulation should be used only by a highly skilled doctor, thoroughly trained in this art, and having the knowledge of both its benefits and dangers

When severe pain, muscle contraction, or both are found in the low back region, the use of pulsed diathermy before manipulation may be desired and appears to make the necessary manipulation less difficult. Fortunately, the greatest percentage of low back pain is at the lower portion of the low back region, whereas the most involved lesion is at the upper portion (thoracolumbar level) of the low back region. With rare exceptions, side-posture manipulation should not be considered during the severely acute stage because of antalgic contraction. When necessary, it should be conducted only by the chiropractor well-versed in the use of side-posture treatment, particularly when used for the reduction of 12th thoracic/1st lumbar lesions. Routine, prone specific manipulation can be done by raising the center section of the adjusting table 3 or 4 inches and raising the lower legs into a slightly flexed position. In most cases, this will be the proper position for specific manipulation to the thoracolumbar area, in acute cases.

> Before the manipulation is conducted, the physician is not to massage, probe, use electrotherapy, or in any other way further activate the anterior or posterior primary rami, or both, which might stimulate muscle reaction

(This recommendation may cause some comment, but it must be remembered that the neural system is subject to stimulation from external forces. When overriding the present abnormal neural reaction, although it may cause temporary muscle relaxation, it may later cause increased muscle response. Such later response can frequently be seen in those cases with secondary lesions. In any event, caution is the best policy.)

The manipulation for a primary disrelated joint should be crisp and done with sufficient force to obtain some movement at the joint. The full range of motion for the joint is not required initially, as further manipulation during follow-up office visits increase the motion until it is normal.

Secondary lesions also require that joint movement be activated. Smaller amounts of joint motion may be all that is required to reduce or control symptoms. In most of these cases, treatment is conducted for symptomatic control, not joint pathological correction.

In most cases, the chiropractor does not adjust a second time for a period of at least 4 to 6 h. There are exceptions. A highly reactive primary lesion that does not release during the first treatment may require additional manipulation in a short period of time, but the doctor should confirm that the correct vertebra is being adjusted. Following treatment, the patient is instructed to return home and rest as much as possible on a couch, lying on his or her side, the back against the back of the couch, legs flexed with a pillow between the knees holding the upper leg on an even level with the hip. Daily treatments are necessary until the acute reactive stage is resolved; the rest periods are reduced as the patient's tolerance allows. The following figures show the best resting positions for most cases suffering with low back/leg pain.

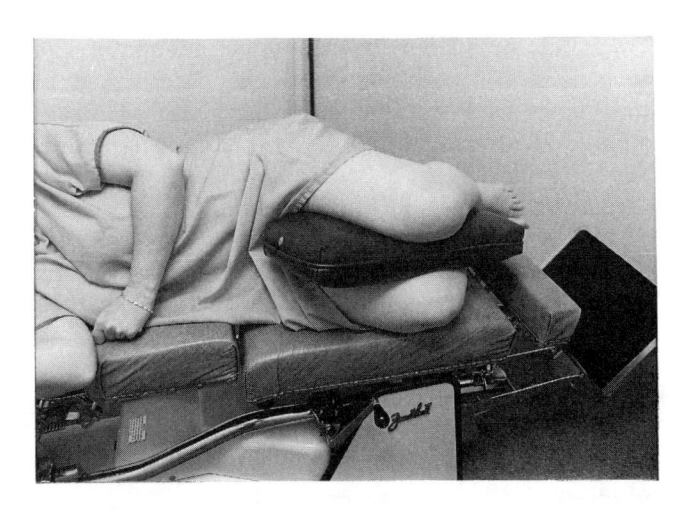

Figure 18–1

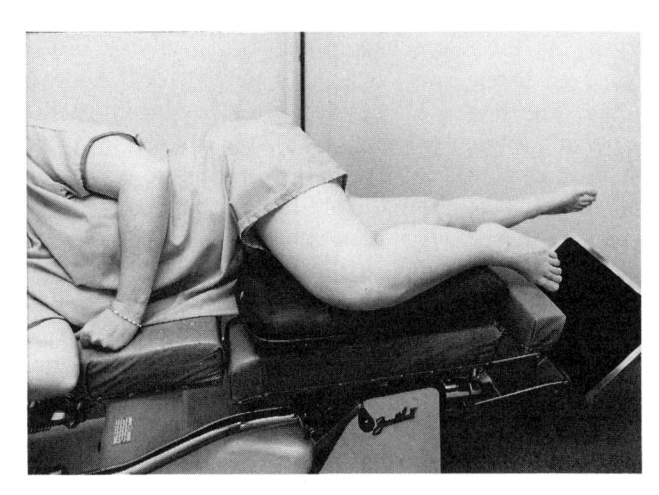

EVALUATION OF TREATMENT FOR LOW BACK/LEG PAIN **103**

Figure 18–2

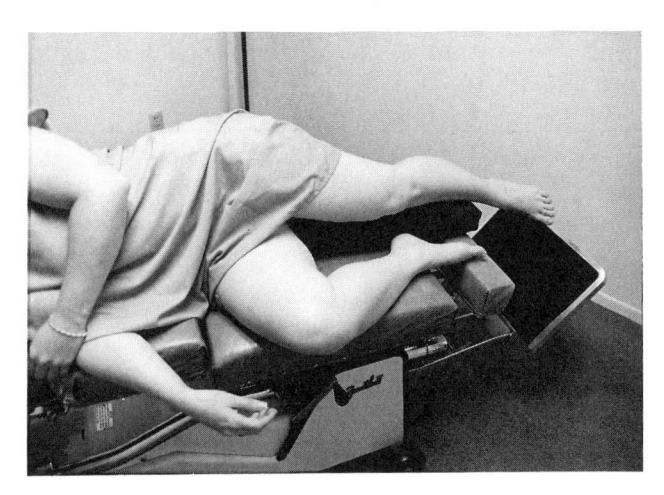

Figure 18–3

If the spinal injury is lower, such as at the 4th or 5th lumbar motor unit and a paraspinal pain syndrome is present with its associated muscle contraction, the doctor follows the above method of treatment until the paraspinal muscle contraction is reduced. Then, the 5th lumbar lesion can be treated with little danger of causing further trauma. In some cases, this may have to be done concurrently. If this situation is present, great care must be taken when treating the 5th lumbar unit. Treatment of a 5th lumbar subluxation/disrelation lesion can be done in the side-posture position as explained later, under torsion roll for 4th or 5th lumbar lesions.

Torsion Roll for the Thoracolumbar Region

When the thoracolumbar or 12th thoracic is so painful that manipulation in the prone position is not recommended, the patient can be treated in the side-posture position. Treatment in this position for the thoracolumbar region is difficult and must be conducted correctly or an increase in pain can be expected. The objective is to produce torsion at the 12th thoracic level, releasing the segmental muscle contraction without causing spinal hyperextension or any thrusts that could increase joint jamming. It can be done in the following manner. The patient lies on his or her side, with the upper leg hanging forward. While facing the patient, the doctor pulls forward the shoulder that is against the table. This places the patient in a position of torsion. The doctor places himself against the table with the patient's top leg between those of the doctor. The wrist is grasped from the arm closest to the table and the hand placed on the upper portion of the other arm. The doctor must ensure that the arms are not crossed (a position that may cause an injury; safety is always essential). The doctor's headward hand is placed over the patient's wrist or hand, and the footward hand positioned at the lumbosacral region, with the doctor's forearm angling downward to the patient's highest hip. Pressure is created just below the doctor's elbow at the medial posterior portion of his or her arm. The middle finger is curled over the spinous process of the vertebra, and a pulling pressure is held at this point. The spinous process contacted will be below the lesion. The doctor is now ready to execute this maneuver. The maneuver consists of three or four short movements, forcing backward with the hand over the wrist and pulling anterior and downward with the hip contact made by the doctor's forearm. The doctor simultaneously pulls in that same direction with the middle finger contacting the spinous process. No more force than that is ever required in all but the most muscular patient. The use of this torsion roll may be required for several treatments. When the segment releases or the segmental rating is reduced on the following visit, treatment is returned to that used in the prone position. The torsion roll is used sparingly and with caution. Figures 18–4 and 18–5 show the basic position.

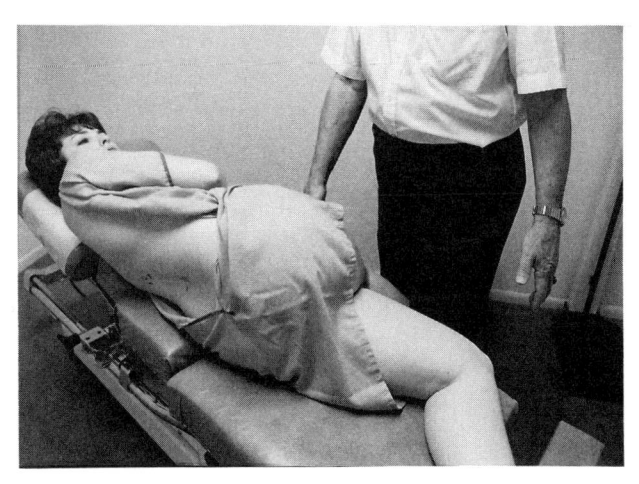

Figure 18–4

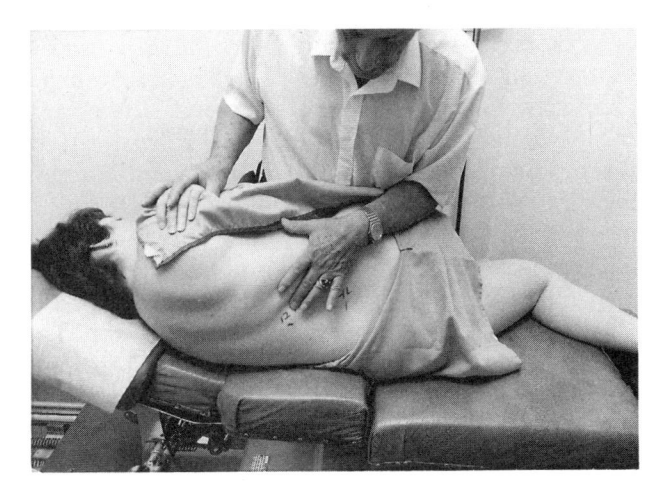

Figure 18-5

Torsion Roll for 4th or 5th Lumbar Vertebra

The torsion roll may be required for cases in which the 5th lumbar is reactive. The index finger contact is made at the 5th lumbar spinous process instead of the 12th thoracic and the procedure is the same, with less torsion required. This maneuver is always followed by manipulation, the patient in the prone position, at the 12th thoracic level. The manipulation need not be heavy (see Fig. 18–6). The patient's leg remains in the same position as shown in Fig. 18–4.

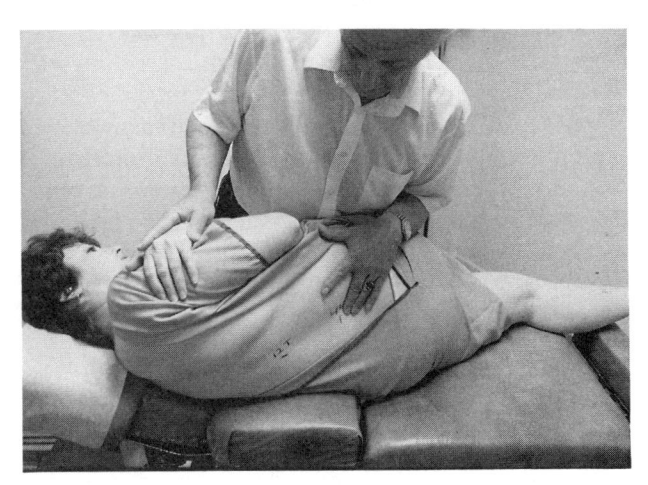

Figure 18-6

Most patients with acute lesions can be manipulated at the 4th or 5th lumbar segments (or both) following the preceding instructions. Some cases, particularly men who are heavily muscled, may require the following method. Because this method of side-posture treatment is capable of producing considerable pressure and torsion, it is not recommended until the chiropractor is well-versed in the lighter type of side-posture treatment.

The patient is positioned as in the previous instructions given for the thoracolumbar region, with the following exception. The patient's upper knee is flexed and that ankle placed on the lower knee. The doctor's footward knee is placed on the patient's knee, enabling the doctor to produce pressure against the patient's knee in a caudalward and downward direction. Holding this pressure, the practitioner slowly forces the patient's upper shoulder backward, and with the footward arm and hand positioned against the patient's upper hip, index finger pulling the 5th lumbar segment, the doctor quickly increases the body torsion while pulling the spinous process with the index finger. The actual torsion motion for the body in this maneuver is very small, but it is an effective method for mobilizing the lumbosacral joint, especially in heavy individuals see Figs. 18–7 and 18–8 showing leg and hand positions. It is also effective in heavy body structures for treatment of the thoracolumbar region (see Fig. 18–9).

Do not use this procedure if hip or knee lesions are present.

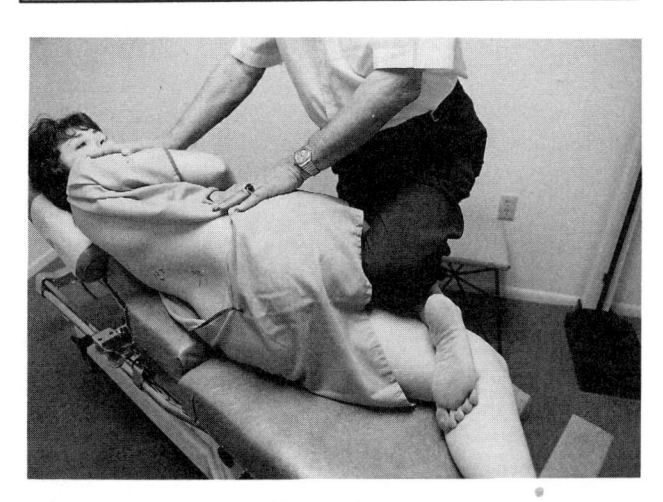

Figure 18-7

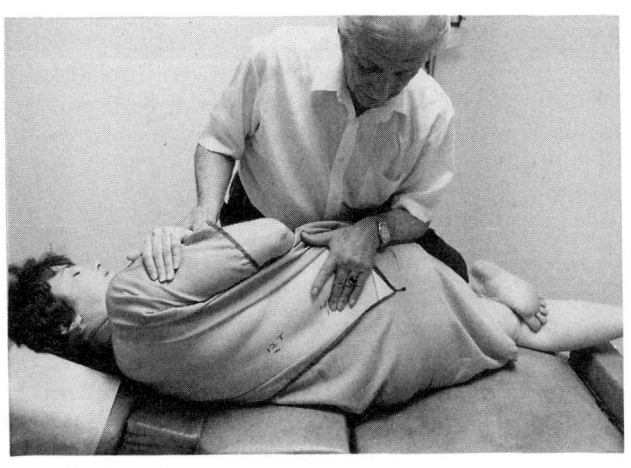

Figure 18-8

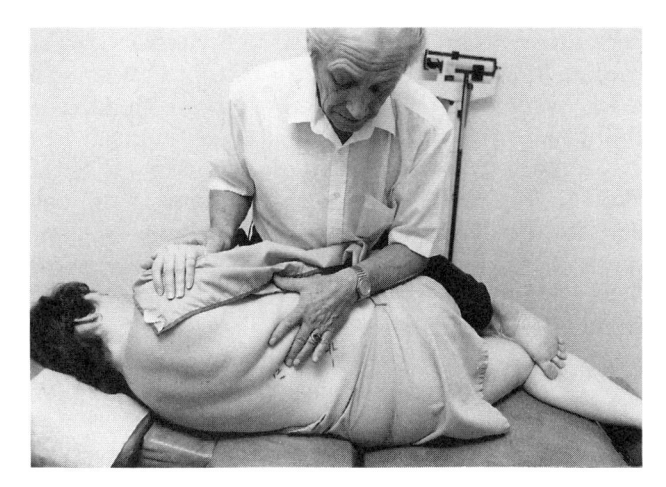

Figure 18–9

The side-posture treatment described should be used only in those cases that cannot be treated in the prone position, or cases in which segmental motion cannot be induced in the prone position. The doctor must be certain that body torque is kept to the minimum required to obtain motion at the spinal segment.

By reducing the primary lesion as soon as possible, the probability is reduced that a secondary spinal lesion will develop from that injury. For those cases in which the injury is more severe, it may aid in preventing unnecessary spreading of the lesion from one segment to another via neural reaction, which may excite tissues that involve other spinal segmental levels.

The secondary spinal lesion already exists in varying degrees within the state where tissues have changed and become pathological. Those tissues that have changed cannot be returned to normal by any form of treatment, but the added subluxation/disrelation lesion that is concurrent with that secondary lesion can in most cases be reduced or controlled. The form of treatment necessary for reduction or control of the reinjured secondary lesion must also be determined by the segmental reaction, patient history, and more important, the type of the basic lesion determined by the x-ray, or other forms of diagnostic equipment. Except for the amount of pain suffered by the patient with a superimposed added injury, there is no pressing need that the secondary subluxation/disrelation lesion per se be reduced, if it is possible to correct or change at all. A reactive primary lesion that is superimposed upon a secondary spinal lesion must be treated by specific manipulation. This treatment has to be accomplished within the framework of the pathological extent of the secondary lesion, and frequently extra care is required. Observation of a secondary spinal lesion via x-ray does not indicate that it is the reactive lesion; this is determined only by the segmental examination.

If the database presented in this text is investigated, it is found that there have been no figures entered for primary and secondary lesions. These figures have not been tabulated at this writing. The author apologizes for this omission, and hopes that these figures will be published in a later publication of this manual. The figures for chronic cases found in this database would of course be secondary lesions and they account for 44% of patients. Acute cases may contain either primary or secondary lesions, and these cases should be separated for statistical references.

The treatment for secondary spinal lesions depends upon the amount of neurological reaction expressed in the form of muscle contraction with resulting pain, and upon how these reactions are associated with the type of underlying joint pathology. It is a rare secondary lesion case, with extreme spinal joint gross pathology, for which specific spinal manipulation is contraindicated. Those constitutional diseases affecting bone, upon which manipulation should not be performed, are well known to the chiropractor skilled in manipulation.

If premanipulation physiotherapy is considered, it should be utilized in a form that does not further excite or traumatize the nerve or nerve groups. For example, the use of sine wave treatment before the manipulation may not be the best procedure. If the subluxation/disrelation lesion is found within severe osteoarthropathy, heavy forms of exercise are not to be recommended. Active exercise for even a minor pathological joint that is reactive and that may cause pain syndromes cannot be considered correct. Although in some cases the pain might be reduced due to exercise, joint pathology could become increased. When the subluxation/disrelation lesion is controlled, gradual mild exercise may be considered and increased slightly if found effective. It is important to always keep in mind that exercise does not correct the state of pathology and thus must be limited.

Ultrasound appears to be very effective in those cases that are resistant to movement, possibly due to associated fibrosis; it can be used at painful muscle attachments. The author has found that lower wattage and longer time exposure appears to be better tolerated by the patient. The use of traction, rollers, and vibrators has little beneficial effect in the treatment of true subluxation/disrelation lesions that are responsible for pain syndromes.

Either prescription or nonprescription pain medication may be desirable during the acute stage, in some cases. Continued use, however, often causes side effects that are worse than the original problem. Nevertheless and more important, medication cannot correct the subluxation/disrelation lesion and can give the patient a sense of security that does not exist. This holds true for other forms of prescription medication used for low back/leg pain cases.

Indicating that a patient might be emotionally disturbed and that this is a cause of low back, pelvic, and leg pain, just does not fit with our present knowledge of these cases. Steady, chronic pain at any one or more of these areas can, without doubt, create frustration, and may cause anger, particularly when the doctor makes statements such as these, "I find no reason for your pain. You should take something to calm you down."; or "Go back to work—that should help"; or "Start on an exercise program."

Then the patient suspects that the doctor does not know what the basic problem is, minimizes the pain being suffered, and then charges a stiff fee. At this point, many individuals become emotionally upset, with good cause, and their consequent annoyance is often carried from physician to physician in the patient's rounds to find the answer to, and subsequent correction of, the pain problem.

The consideration of surgical intervention should not be taken lightly. Even the use of injections into or near the pathological joint, although offering immediate relief, may further damage the injured tissue, aggravate the neural system, or both. This form of treatment can also give the patient a false sense of security, allowing the patient to further damage the joint with activities that should not be done. Radical surgery certainly carries a greater responsibility for the physician than does conservative treatment, and should be considered only as a last resort. Before this type of treatment is utilized, the segmental reaction must be highly reactive at the level considered for surgery. If it is not reactive, further study should be conducted and the diagnosis might well be questioned.

The latest research in low back leg pain, published in the European edition of *Spine*,* has made several observations. This research was conducted in Quebec, Canada. No member of the chiropractic profession or chiropractic college was found among the executive staff or members of this task force on low back/leg pain. It appears that one chiropractor may have served in an advisory capacity.

The preliminary observation states that the terminology and nosology regarding spinal disorders are neither standardized nor validated. (The healing arts have been aware of this problem for many years, with little progress in making a change.)

They state in their general conclusions that the etiologic diagnosis of spinal disorders is difficult because the physical signs and symptoms often have little specificity. (The specificity *is* there, but diagnostic and examination procedures were previously absent. The procedures followed in this book should aid in correcting this deficit.)

The following are some of the points they felt required special mention:

1. They state in general that the symptoms of acute pain in the lumbar, dorsal, and cervical regions tend to resolve spontaneously. (The author believes that it is true in some cases, but may also lead to the secondary subluxation.)
2. They also indicate that obligatory bed rest in low back pain, without significant radiation of pain, is not required. When prescribed, only 2 days are required for low back pain, and 7 days for cervical pain. They state that prolonged bed rest can have adverse effects.
3. They feel that surgery is not indicated for low back pain when an anatomical disorder is not objectively demonstrated.
4. Their findings indicate that surgery, including chemonucleolysis, should not be performed until conservative treatment has failed.
5. Their findings have shown that return to work is not contraindicated even if residual chronic pain is present. They feel that work may be therapeutic.
6. One important comment made was that muscle spasm is mainly protective in nature. The author does not disagree with that.

They have discussed a variety of treatment, including manipulation, which they recommend as effective. They state, however, that all the studies were conducted in a medical or osteopathic milieu; there were no properly controlled chiropractic studies on this subject.

It is doubtful that every doctor within the healing arts will take the time or have the desire to become competent in the diagnosis of low back, pelvic, and leg pain cases. Probably the best that can be hoped for is that the specific differential diagnosis and treatment for low back cases will ultimately become a specialty field. The average practitioner should nevertheless have at least some knowledge in this field although aware of his or her limitations.

---

* Members of the Quebec task force on low back leg pain: Treatment of activity-related spinal disorders. *Spine* 12 (7s):s22, 1987.

Chapter 19

Database on Low Back, Pelvic, and Leg Pain

Clinical research for low back, pelvic, and leg pain must be expressed in the form of a database in order for each segment of that information to become of value within its relationship to the total knowledge of these conditions.

This database should and will be added to, as each addition will update and give information that will further increase our total knowledge of low back, pelvic, and leg pain cases.

The following database is shown specifically for use as a condensed guide that can aid in the further evaluation of these cases.

The author has also placed graphic illustrations below for each syndrome and group for rapid evaluation.

SINGLE PAIN SYNDROME CASES

These statistics were taken from only those cases in which pain was found in a single pain syndrome area (an area supplied by only one nerve or nerve group).

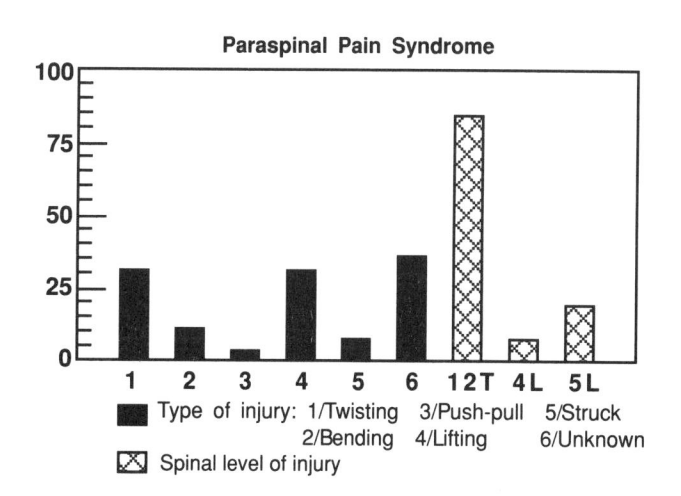

1. *Paraspinal:* 42% of all single pain syndrome cases (number of cases: 176)

The most frequent level of injury was the 12th thoracic–1st lumbar (posterior primary rami).

Incidence
Male	63%	Female	37%
Acute	66%	Chronic	34%

Type of injury
Twisting	29%	Lifting	27%
Bending	11%	Struck	4%
Push–pull	2%	Unknown	34%

Spinal level injured
12th thoracic	86%	5th lumbar	22%
4th lumbar	5%		

Spinal levels treated by specific manipulation
12th thoracic	84%	5th lumbar	25%
4th lumbar	5%		

Twelve patients of this group were classified as unknown, tourists, transients, etc. Ten patients of this group did not begin treatment, or discontinued treatment.

Results from treatment in 154 cases are noted below.

Released asymptomatic
Acute	33	Chronic	14

Good: slight discomfort to pain free—short of release
Acute	63	Chronic	41

Fair: postsurgical or severe pathology
Acute	2	Chronic	0

Poor
Acute	1	Chronic	0

Paraspinal Pain Syndrome

Type of injury: 1/Twisting 3/Push-pull 5/Struck
2/Bending 4/Lifting 6/Unknown
Spinal level of injury

Paraspinal Pain Syndrome

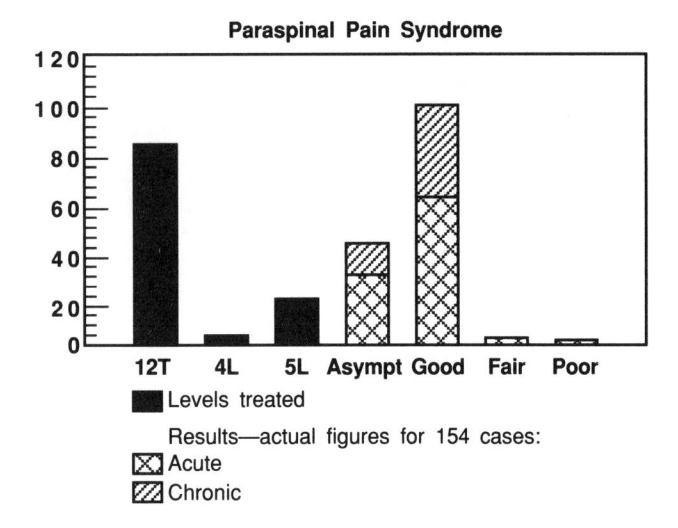

Results—actual figures for 154 cases:
- Acute
- Chronic

2. *Lumbar:* 28% of all single pain syndrome cases (number of cases: 116)

The most frequent level of injury was the 5th lumbar (posterior primary rami).

Incidence
Male	68%	Female	32%
Acute	77%	Chronic	21%

Type of injury
Lifting	30%	Twisting	21%
Bending	12%	Falls	9%
Struck	2%	Push–pull	4%
Unknown	28%		

Spinal levels injured
12th thoracic	39%	5th lumbar	70%
4th lumbar	13%		

Spinal levels treated by specific manipulation
12th thoracic	67%	5th lumbar	65%
4th lumbar	12%		

Twelve patients in this group are listed as unknown. Eleven patients did not start, or discontinued.
Results from treatment in 93 cases are noted below.

Released asymptomatic
Acute	21	Chronic	0

Good
Acute	50	Chronic	15

Fair
Acute	3	Chronic	3

Poor
Acute	0	Chronic	1

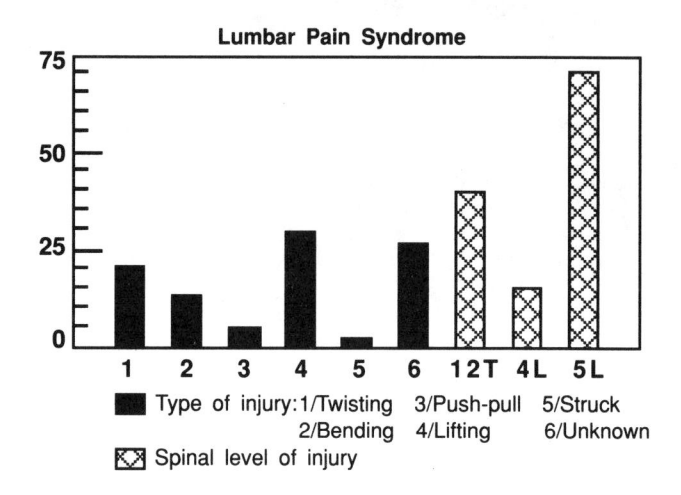

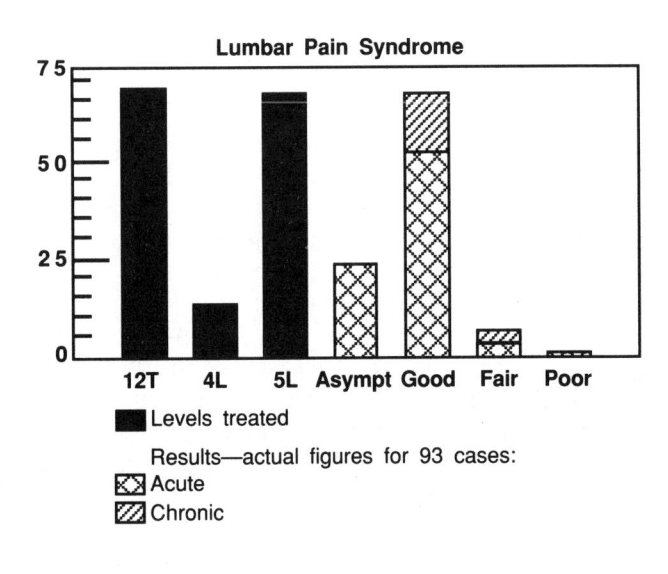

Lumbar Pain Syndrome

Type of injury: 1/Twisting 2/Bending 3/Push-pull 4/Lifting 5/Struck 6/Unknown
Spinal level of injury

Lumbar Pain Syndrome

Levels treated
Results—actual figures for 93 cases:
- Acute
- Chronic

3. *Gluteal:* 3% of all single pain syndrome cases (number of cases: 11)

The most frequent level of injury was the 12th thoracic (posterior primary rami)

Incidence
Male	45%	Female	55%
Acute	91%	Chronic	9%

Type of injury
Lifting	27%	Twisting	27%
Bending	9%	Fall	9%
Push–pull	9%	Unknown	27%

Spinal levels injured
12th thoracic	82%	5th lumbar	18%
4th lumbar	9%		

Spinal levels treated by specific manipulation
12th thoracic	91%	5th lumbar	27%
4th lumbar	27%		

Three patients in this group are listed as unknown.

Results from treatment in 8 cases are noted below.

Released asymptomatic
Acute	1	Chronic	1

Good
Acute	6	Chronic	0

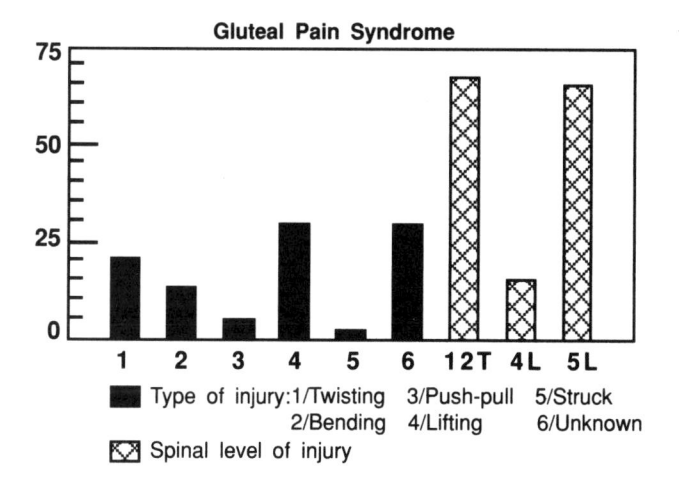

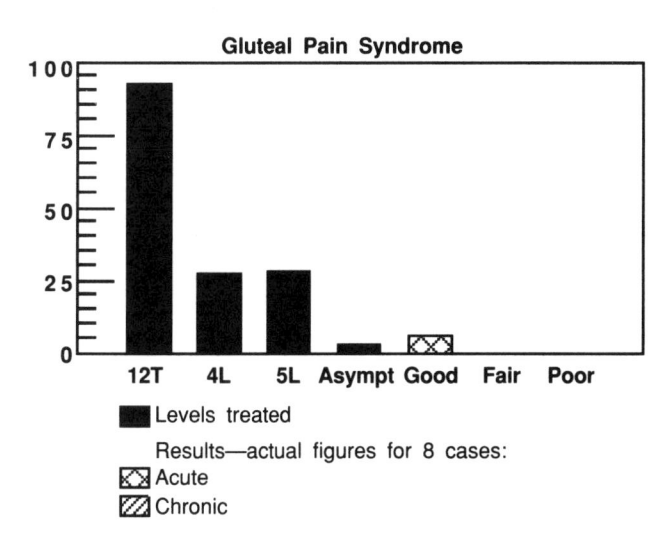

Gluteal Pain Syndrome [bar chart showing type of injury and spinal level of injury: 1/Twisting, 2/Bending, 3/Push-pull, 4/Lifting, 5/Struck, 6/Unknown; spinal levels 12T, 4L, 5L]

Gluteal Pain Syndrome [bar chart showing levels treated (12T, 4L, 5L) and results (Asympt, Good, Fair, Poor) — actual figures for 8 cases: Acute, Chronic]

4. *Thomas:* 4% of all single pain syndrome cases (number of cases: 15)

The most common level of injury was the 12th thoracic (anterior primary rami).

Incidence
Male	40%	Female	60%
Acute	80%	Chronic	20%

Type of injury
Lifting	27%	Bending	13%
Twisting	13%	Fall	7%
Struck	7%	Push–pull	7%
Unknown	33%		

Spinal levels injured
12th thoracic	80%	5th lumbar	27%
4th lumbar	7%		

Spinal level treated by specific manipulation
12th thoracic	87%	5th lumbar	20%
4th lumbar	7%		

Two patients in this group are listed as unknown.

Results from treatment in 13 cases are noted below.

Released asymptomatic
Acute	2	Chronic	0

Good
Acute	8	Chronic	3

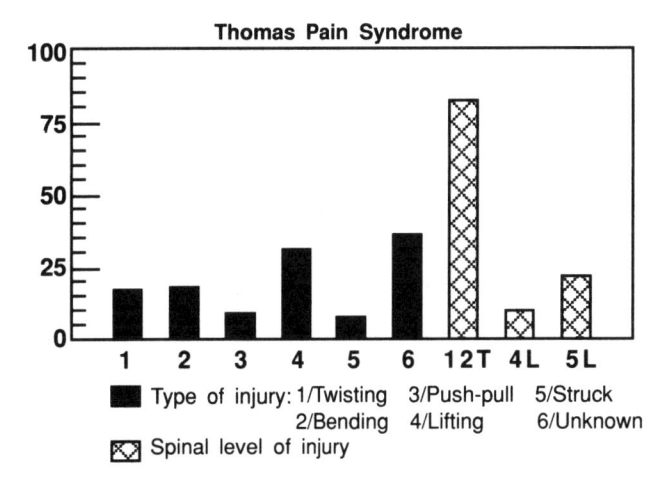

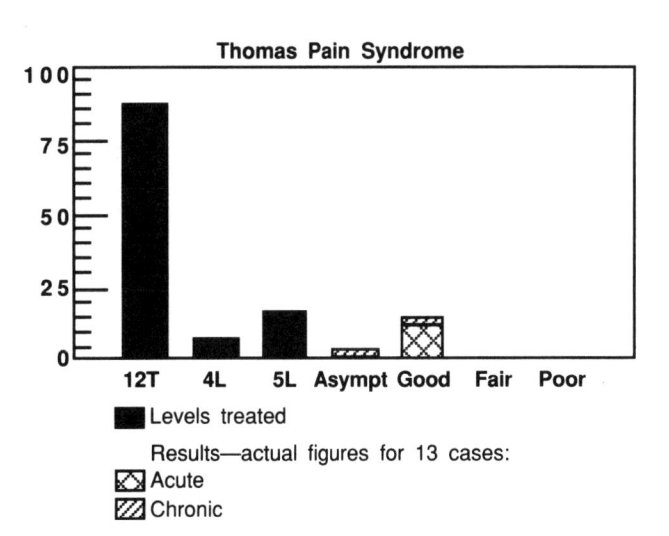

Thomas Pain Syndrome [bar chart showing type of injury and spinal level of injury: 1/Twisting, 2/Bending, 3/Push-pull, 4/Lifting, 5/Struck, 6/Unknown; spinal levels 12T, 4L, 5L]

Thomas Pain Syndrome [bar chart showing levels treated (12T, 4L, 5L) and results (Asympt, Good, Fair, Poor) — actual figures for 13 cases: Acute, Chronic]

5. *Inguinal:* 4% of all single pain syndrome cases (number of cases: 15)

The most common level of injury was the 12th thoracic (anterior primary rami).

Incidence
Male	60%	Female	40%
Acute	53%	Chronic	47%

Type of injury
Lifting	13%	Twisting	47%
Bending	7%	Fall	1%
Struck	7%	Unknown	40%

Spinal levels injured
12th thoracic	100%	5th lumbar	13%

Spinal levels treated by specific manipulation
12th thoracic	100%	5th lumbar	13%

One patient in this group is listed as unknown. Results of treatment in 14 cases are noted below.

Released asymptomatic
Acute	3	Chronic	2
Good	4	Chronic	3
Fair	0	Chronic	2

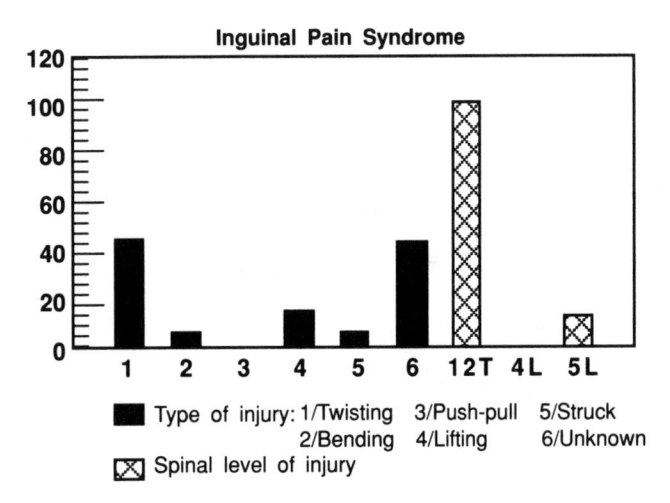

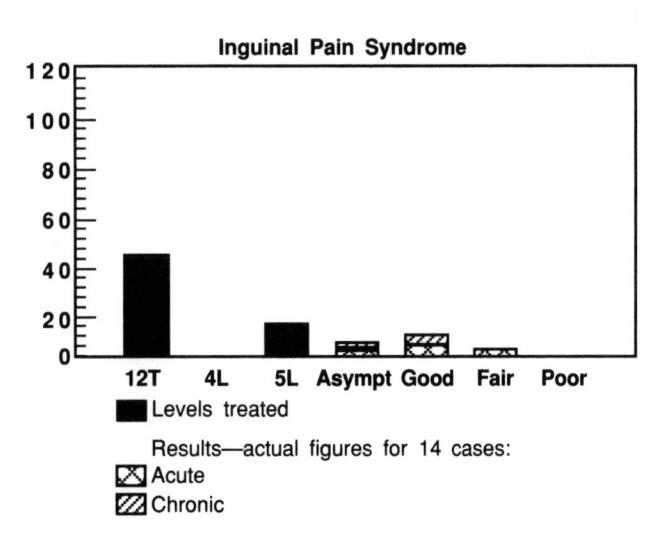

Inguinal Pain Syndrome (bar chart: Type of injury: 1/Twisting, 2/Bending, 3/Push-pull, 4/Lifting, 5/Struck, 6/Unknown; Spinal level of injury)

Inguinal Pain Syndrome (bar chart: Levels treated at 12T, 4L, 5L; Results—actual figures for 14 cases: Acute, Chronic — Asympt, Good, Fair, Poor)

6. *Anterior Femoral:* 7% of all single pain syndrome cases (number of cases: 29)

The most common level of injury was the 12th thoracic (anterior primary rami).

Incidence
Male	55%	Female	45%
Acute	48%	Chronic	52%

Type of injury
Lifting	17%	Twisting	21%
Bending	17%	Fall	7%
Push-pull	3%	Unknown	52%

Spinal levels injured
12th thoracic	100%	5th lumbar	14%
4th lumbar	3%		

Spinal levels treated by specific manipulation
12th thoracic	100%	5th lumbar	10%
4th lumbar	3%		

Three patients in this group are listed as unknown. Results from treatment in 26 cases are noted below.

Released asymptomatic
Acute	5	Chronic	1
Good			
Acute	7	Chronic	11
Poor			
Acute	1	Chronic	1

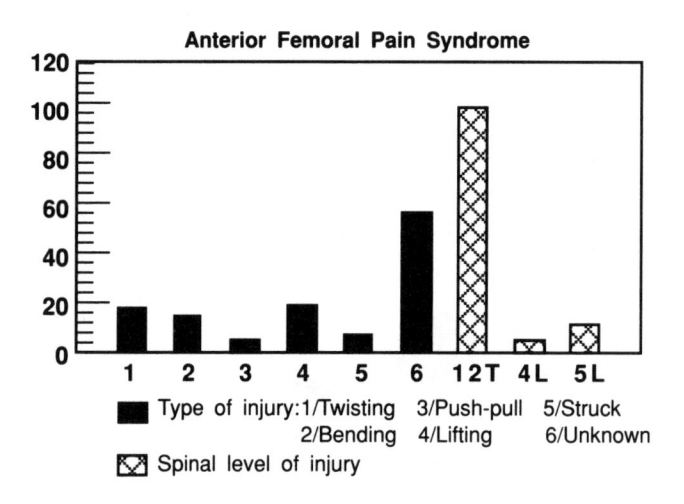

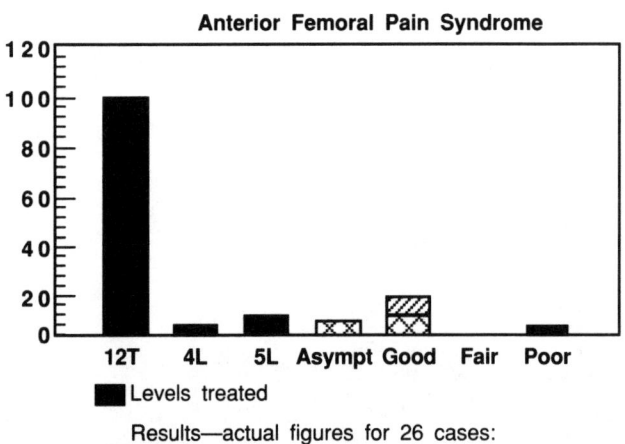

Anterior Femoral Pain Syndrome (bar chart: Type of injury: 1/Twisting, 2/Bending, 3/Push-pull, 4/Lifting, 5/Struck, 6/Unknown; Spinal level of injury)

Anterior Femoral Pain Syndrome (bar chart: Levels treated at 12T, 4L, 5L; Results—actual figures for 26 cases: Acute, Chronic — Asympt, Good, Fair, Poor)

7. *Lateral Femoral:* 7% of all single pain syndrome cases (number of cases: 28)

The most common level of injury was the 12th thoracic (anterior primary rami).

Incidence
Male	50%	Female	50%
Acute	46%	Chronic	46%
Unknown	8%		

Type of injury
Lifting	11%	Twisting	4%
Bending	14%	Fall	4%
Unknown	75%		

Spinal levels injured
12th thoracic	92%	5th lumbar	11%
4th lumbar	4%		

Spinal levels treated by specific manipulation
12th thoracic	100%	5th lumbar	14%
4th lumbar	4%		

Three patients in this group are listed as unknown. Seven patients terminated treatment or did not begin.

Results from treatment in 18 cases are noted below.

Released asymptomatic
Acute	3	Chronic	3

Good
Acute	5	Chronic	7

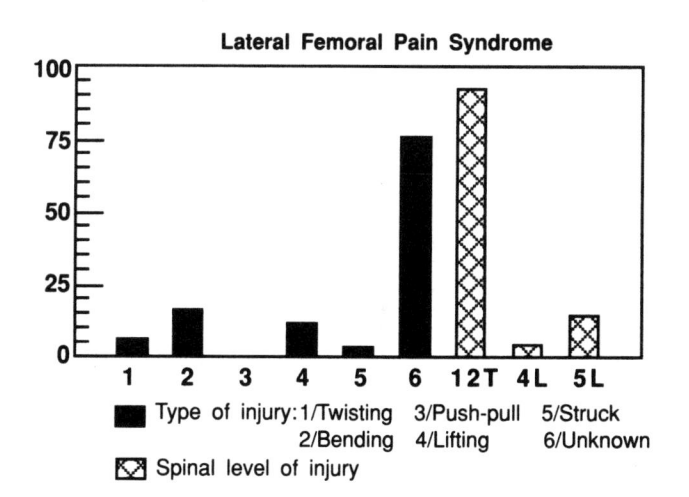

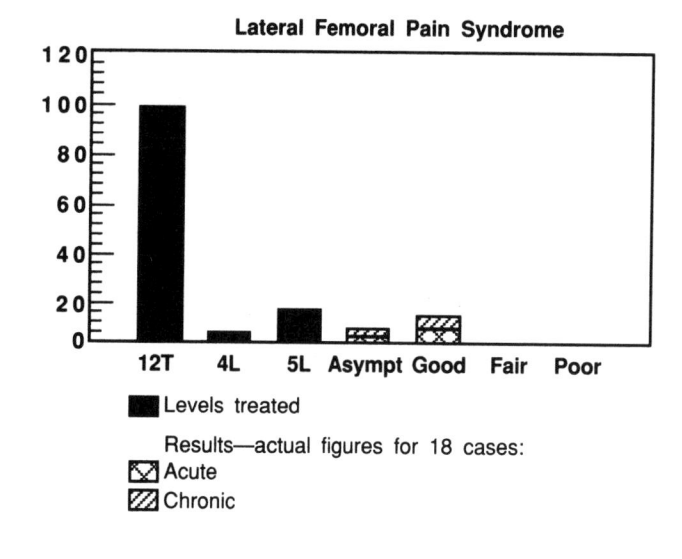

8. *Posterior Femoral:* 6% of all single pain syndrome cases (number of cases: 27).

The most common level of injury was the 5th lumbar (anterior primary rami).

Incidence
Male	56%	Female	44%
Acute	56%	Chronic	44%

Type of injury
Lifting	11%	Twisting	22%
Bending	22%	Fall	11%
Struck	7%	Unknown	48%

Spinal level injured
12th thoracic	52%	5th lumbar	62%
4th lumbar	11%		

Spinal levels treated by specific manipulation
12th thoracic	56%	5th lumbar	74%
4th lumbar	7%		

Three patients in this group are unknown. Two patients did not begin treatment.

Results from treatment in 22 cases are noted below.

Released asymptomatic
Acute	7	Chronic	2

Good
Acute	4	Chronic	6

Fair
Acute	0	Chronic	2

Poor
Acute	1	Chronic	0

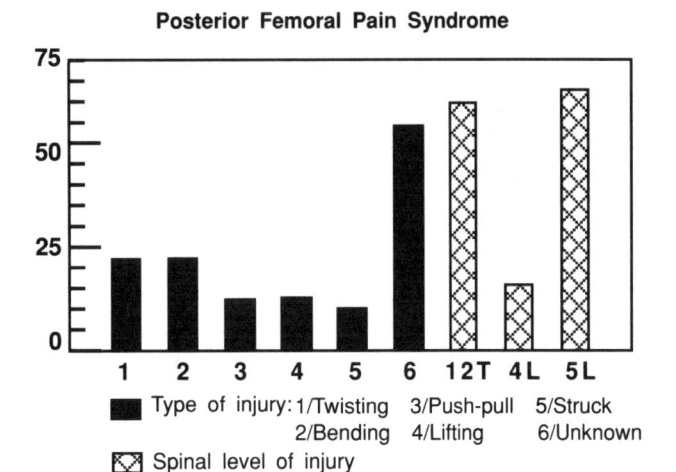

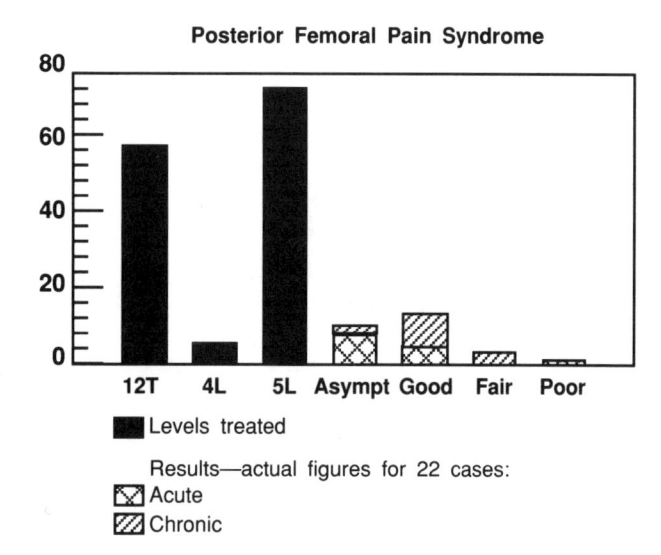

Posterior Femoral Pain Syndrome

(chart: bars for types of injury 1-6 and spinal levels 12T, 4L, 5L)

Type of injury: 1/Twisting 3/Push-pull 5/Struck
2/Bending 4/Lifting 6/Unknown
Spinal level of injury

Posterior Femoral Pain Syndrome

(chart: 12T, 4L, 5L, Asympt, Good, Fair, Poor)

Levels treated

Results—actual figures for 22 cases:
Acute
Chronic

The methods used to gather the preceding information for single pain syndrome areas must be known to the physician before the composite pain syndromes can be understood and treated with any assurance of success. Composite pain syndromes are those cases in which pain is found in more than one pain syndrome area.

Composite syndromes are found in 27% of all low back/leg pain cases. Patients with two syndromes account for 21% of all cases. Patients with three or more syndromes are found in 6% of all cases.

The analysis of the 27% for composite syndromes is as follows:

- Combined lumbar and paraspinal are found in 10% of the composite syndromes.
- The anterior femoral with one other syndrome amounts to 23%.
- The lateral femoral with one other syndrome is 14%.
- The posterior femoral with one other syndrome totals 16%.

The total number of posterior femoral syndromes, found in the composite 27%, amounts to only 24% of that figure. Each combination could be analyzed down statistically but no pattern, to date, has been shown.

The analysis on all double pain syndromes is as follows:

DOUBLE PAIN SYNDROMES

(Number of cases: 121)

Incidence
Male	52%	Female	48%
Acute	59%	Chronic	41%

Type of injury
Lifting	29%	Twisting	17%
Bending	11%	Unknown	43%

Spinal level injured
12th thoracic	96%	5th lumbar	24%
4th lumbar	12%		

Spinal level treated by specific manipulation
12th thoracic	83%	5th lumbar	35%
4th lumbar	9%		

Four patients terminated treatment or did not start in this group. Nineteen patients in this group are unknown.

Results from treatment in 98 cases are noted below.

Released asymptomatic
Acute	24	Chronic	11

Good
Acute	33	Chronic	25

Fair
Acute	0	Chronic	3

Poor
Acute	1	Chronic	1

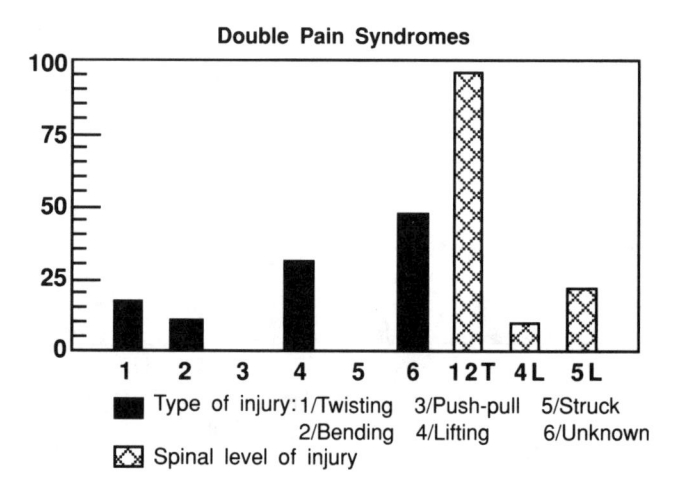

Double Pain Syndromes

(chart: bars for types of injury 1-6 and spinal levels 12T, 4L, 5L)

Type of injury: 1/Twisting 3/Push-pull 5/Struck
2/Bending 4/Lifting 6/Unknown
Spinal level of injury

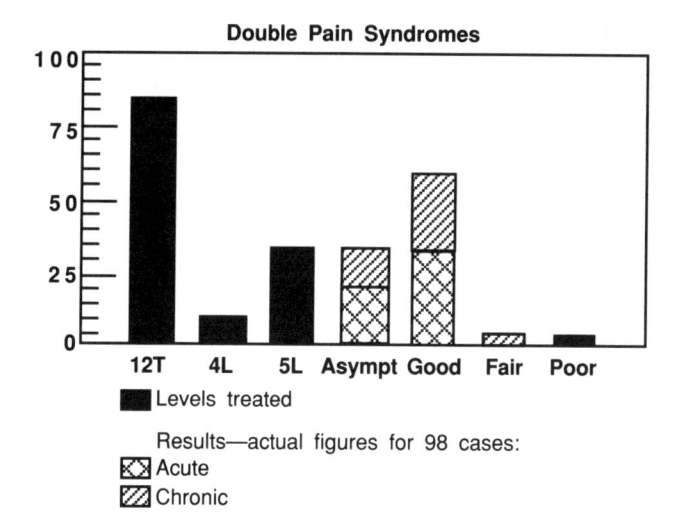

THREE OR MORE PAIN SYNDROMES

(Number of cases: 34)

Incidence
Male	44%	Female	56%
Acute	35%	Chronic	65%

Type of injury
Lifting	26%	Twisting	3%
Bending	15%	Fall	15%
Struck	6%	Push–pull	3%
Unknown	44%		

Spinal levels injured
12th thoracic	89%	5th lumbar	15%
4th lumbar	9%		

Spinal levels treated by specific manipulation
12th thoracic	95%	5th lumbar	27%
4th lumbar	15%		

Eight patients in this group are listed as unknown.

Results from treatment in 26 cases are noted below.

Released asymptomatic
Acute	3	Chronic	1

Good
Acute	3	Chronic	14

Fair
Acute	1	Chronic	2

Poor
Acute	1	Chronic	1

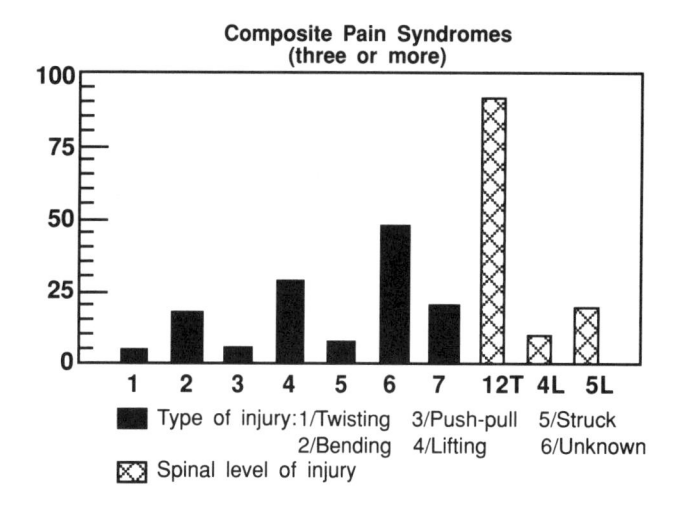

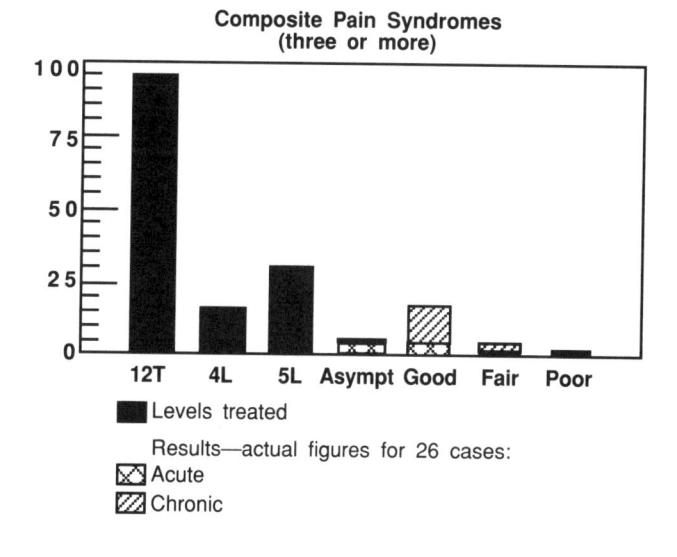

TOTALS FOR THE 8 PRIMARY SYNDROMES

(Number of cases: 417)

Incidence
Male	55%	Female	45%
Acute	65%	Chronic	34%
Unknown	1%		

Type of injury
Lifting	20%	Twisting	23%
Bending	13%	Struck	5%
Push–pull	5%	Fall	4%
Unknown	42%		

The most common levels of injury: 12th thoracic for 6 syndromes, 5th lumbar for 2 syndromes.

Spinal levels injured
12th thoracic	78%	5th lumbar	30%
4th lumbar	7%		

Spinal levels treated by specific manipulation
12th thoracic	87%	5th lumbar	31%
4th lumbar	9%		

Results from treatment in 348 cases are noted below.

Released asymptomatic
Acute   75   Chronic   23
Good
Acute   147   Chronic   86
Fair
Acute   5   Chronic   7
Poor
Acute   3   Chronic   2

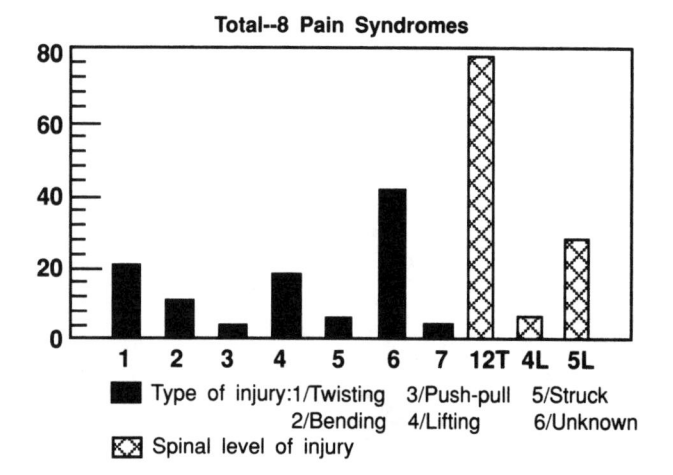

The most common level of injury was the 12th thoracic.

Spinal levels injured
12th thoracic   93%   5th lumbar   20%
4th lumbar   11%
Spinal levels treated by specific manipulation
12th thoracic   89%   5th lumbar   31%
4th lumbar   12%

Results from treatment in 124 cases are noted below.

Released asymptomatic
Acute   27   Chronic   12
Good
Acute   36   Chronic   39
Fair
Acute   1   Chronic   5
Poor
Acute   2   Chronic   2

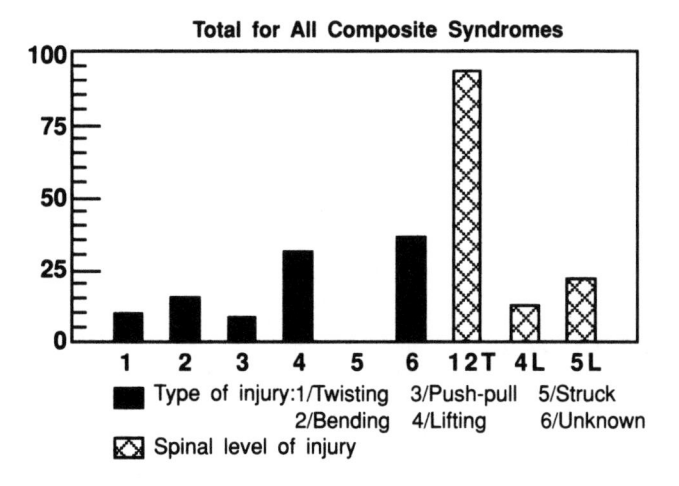

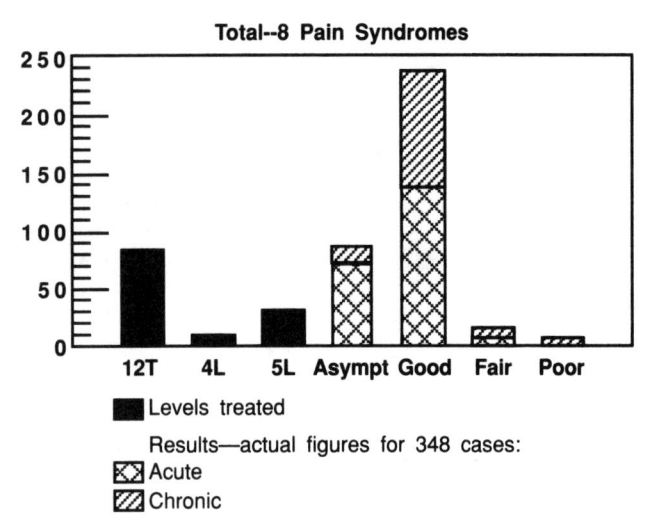

TOTALS FOR COMPOSITE SYNDROMES

(Number of cases: 155)

Incidence
Male   48%   Female   52%
Acute   47%   Chronic   53%
Type of injury
Lifting   28%   Twisting   10%
Bending   13%   Fall   15%
Unknown   43%

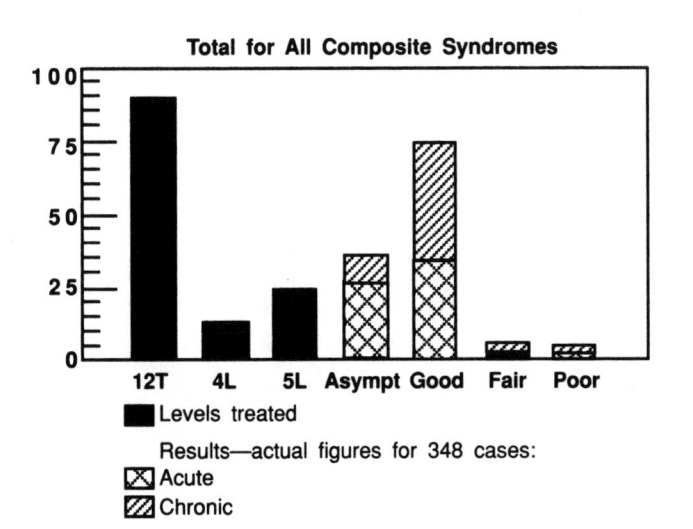

TOTALS FOR ALL SYNDROMES

It is of vital importance that we do not lose sight of the individual pain syndrome, but for the complete picture, let us now combine all cases.

(Number of cases: 572)

Incidence
Male	52%	Female	48%
Acute	56%	Chronic	44%

Type of injuries
Lifting	24%	Twisting	17%
Bending	13%	Fall	10%
Unknown	43%		

The most frequent reactive spinal levels responsible for pain, found in all pain syndromes during spinal segmental examination procedures, was the 12th thoracic and 5th lumbar joints, respectively.

Spinal levels injured
12th thoracic	84%	5th lumbar	25%
4th lumbar	9%		

Spinal levels treated by specific manipulation
12th thoracic	88%	5th lumbar	31%
4th lumbar	11%		

Results from treatment in 472 cases are noted below.

Released asymptomatic
Pain free	137

Good
Near pain free—ready to release	308

Fair
Reduction of symptoms (permanent disability)	18

Poor
Most postsurgical or severe pathology	9

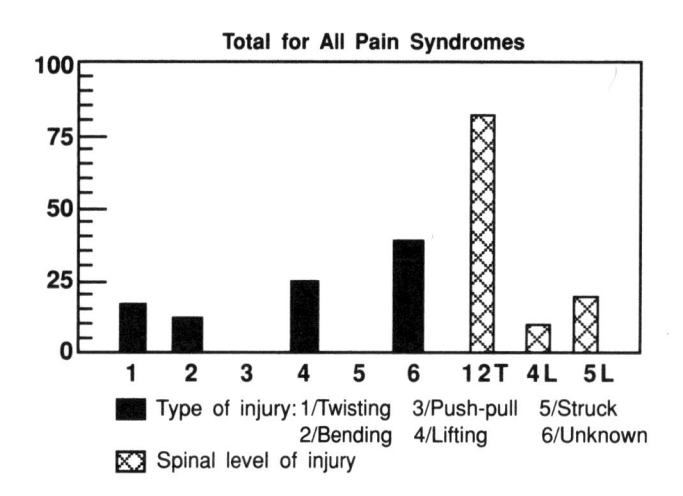

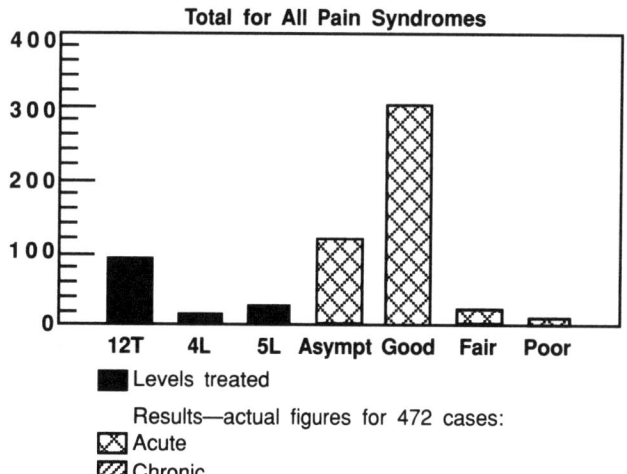

Appendix A

Bibliography for Low Back, Pelvic, and Leg Pain

There is a great deal of information related to low back/leg pain and its causes that has been printed over the years. This information is found in a variety of texts, papers, journals, and scientific reports. If the information that has value is separated from the remainder one arrives at a better understanding of spinal lesions and their syndromes. It is unfortunate that most of this valid information is buried in reports; in many cases it does not surface again for years until it is refound or rewritten about, and only then when its relationship with newer work is confirmed. Even basic information in qualified texts is often ignored until its validity has been reestablished when it is correlated with more up-to-date research findings. This situation probably cannot be criticized as it acts as a system of checks and balances. It is time, however, that some of this information should be condensed and made available to those physicians who must diagnose and treat low back, pelvic, and leg pain cases.

There are many occasions in dealing with members of the insurance industry, medicare, other third-party payors, and attorneys, when the diagnosis, description of pathology, length of treatment, kind of treatment, and so on, is challenged. When this occurs, some scientific or acceptable backup information is desirable. Most practitioners rarely take the time to record information they read that might be of value to them, and they frequently throw informative papers, journals, and so forth, in a pile hoping that they will organize it at a later date. Most frequently, this never happens; when material is needed it is seldom found, or a flurry of time-consuming activity is created in the pursuit of the information. The usual results are the discovery of material that is less than desired.

This Appendix will fulfill the need for substantial data by making support material easily available as a bibliography, and also associating the data with a short explanation of the material in question. Thus, the reader is provided with the range of basic accessible information, and may be prompted to investigate the original work. The information in this Appendix is not meant to take the place of the original articles, nor does it offer a total description of the original work. It functions only as a guide and a point of reference for those interested, and helps to inform the reader that information regarding the subject is available.

The bibliographies are separated in order to provide information related to the joint or nerve lesion because, under certain conditions, both are not present. Should references to both type of lesions be desired, they can be combined yet remain distinct.

New additions can easily be added to these lists for further and ready references. In order to associate the pain syndrome with the spinal joint, nerve lesion, or both, the following section gives references for this connection.

1. SPINAL JOINT LESION

A spinal joint lesion is *Any pathological or traumatic discontinuity of tissue, or loss of function of a part (Dorland's Illustrated Medical Dictionary)*

Of prime importance related to low back, pelvic, and leg pain is the lesion or lesions that cause this condition. It is well-known that gross pathology can cause pain symptoms; however, it is also known that patients may have gross spinal pathological lesions and never suffer from pain symptoms until an injury precipitates the pain.

The term "subluxation" is a limited descriptive term coined to differentiate the relationship that exists between the facets of one vertebra and the facets of the adjacent vertebra, from a luxation in which this relationship is totally destroyed. It is, however, the basis for a variety of lesions that fit within this classification. The author prefers to use the term subluxation/disrelation lesion because it identifies the perimeters of location and degree, and also indicates that a joint or soft-tissue disrelation lesion is present.

Because the term gives a basic perimeter for those varied spinal lesions causing low back/leg pain, there is no real need to dispense with it. In fact, used as a basic classification, it aids both the chiropractor and third parties to better understand the extent of the lesion. When considered in this light, it can be used effectively by giving the most important perimeter and the general location of the spinal lesion without a lengthy narrative report that might be misunderstood. The following bibliography offers some information regarding this generic lesion. Although the pathologies are not named a subluxation/disrelation lesion in each case, they are still lesions, less than a luxation (subluxation).

Consider that this lesion, the subluxation, has been known and discussed over a period of many years and has withstood this long duration of time.

1. Hadley LA: Intervertebral joint subluxation, bony impingement and foramen encroachment with nerve root changes. *AJR* 26(3):377, 1951
   This article shows x-rays of spinal nerve degeneration found in cadavers as a final result of a subluxation.
2. American Medical Association: *Guides to the Evaluation of Permanent Impairment,* 3rd ed. Chicago, American Medical Association, 1988;p.47
   The subluxation is listed as a spinal lesion and rated for permanent impairment.
3. Farfan HF: The use of mechanical etiology to determine the efficacy of active intervention in single joint lumbar intervertebral joint problems. *Spine* 10(4): 350, 1985
   Injuries to the spinal joint resulting from forced axial rotation and lateral flexion under torsional loads are discussed.
4. Brantingham JW: A survey of literature regarding the behavior, pathology, ideologies and nomenclature of the chiropractic lesion. *Journal of Chiropractic* 22(8):p.65, 1985
   Dr. Bantingham discusses how a true subluxation may cause restricted intervertebral motion causing joint pathology with resulting pain.
5. Farfan HF: The use of mechanical etiology to determine the efficacy of active intervention in single joint lumbar intervertebral joint problems. *Spine* 10(4): 350, 1985
   The mechanism of spinal joint failure is explained.
6. Farfan HF: The use of mechanical etiology to determine the efficacy of active intervention in single joint lumbar intervertebral joint problems. *Spine* 10(4): 350, 1985
   This report indicates how torsion injuries, joint subluxation, may develop into joint traumatic arthritis, and how joint injuries may result in joint failure.
7. Wood L: Acute locked facet syndrome and its treatment by manipulation under local periarticular anesthesia—Part 1: Clinical perspective and pilot study proposal. *JMPT* 7(4):211, 1984
   Wood discusses the locking of the spinal joint by the subluxation with muscle spasm, and how this locking may result in osteoarthritis.
8. Good AB: Spinal joint blocking. *JMPT* 8(1):1, 1985
   This is a fine article discussing spinal joint blocking, pain, and muscle spasm.
9. Foreman SM: Ossification of posterior longitudinal ligament—a cause of spinal stenosis. *JMPT* 7(1):253
   A discussion on how ossification of the posterior longitudinal ligament is one cause of spinal stenosis.
10. Dishman R: Review of the literature supporting a scientific basis for the chiropractic subluxation complex. *JMPT* 8(3):163, 1985
    Dr. Dishman indicates the presence of fibrils, fibrosis, and scar tissue found resulting from joint injury, and that a long period of treatment may be required due to these tissue changes.

2. SPINAL LESIONS AND PATHOLOGY (NERVES)

In order that the spinal lesion, gross or subluxation, be able to produce pain either close to the spine or away from the spine, it must involve the nervous system that carries the pain fibers. In spinal joint lesions, injury or reaction to those nerve or nerve groups must occur either at the spinal joint or intervertebral foramen from reactive tissues that might be associated with the injury, joint contusion, or from tissues activated by the neural reaction that is a consequence of injury or joint pathology. The following references give us an insight into this neurological maze.

1. Dishman R: Review of the literature supporting a scientific basis for the chiropractic subluxation complex. *JMPT* 8(3):163, 1985
   This article describes how biochemical changes occur due to the lack of spinal joint movement, and discusses the chemical changes at that area affecting the spinal nerve.
2. Rydevik B, Brown M, Lundborg G: Pathoanatomy

and pathophysiology of nerve root compression. *Spine* 9(1):7, 1984

This is a fine article discussing the pathophysiology and pathoanatomy of nerve root compression. The author also states that compression of the nerve root ganglion may produce repetitive firing of the nerve causing pain, and that chronic nerve compression causes neural excitability, resulting in pain and possible paresthesia.

3. Kirkaldy-Willis WH: *A Scientific Approach: Managing Low Back Pain*, 2nd ed. New York, Churchill Livingstone, 1988;p.93

This work discusses nerve entrapment, nerve disfunction, herniation, stenosis, and spinal joint instability.

4. Wood L: Acute locked facet syndrome and its treatment by manipulation under local periarticular anesthesia—Part 1: Clinical perspective and pilot study proposal. *JMPT* 7(4):211, 1984

The sinuvertebral nerve is discussed in this article, and it is shown that its influence does not appear to extend beyond the spinal canal.

5. Wood L: Acute locked facet syndrome and its treatment by manipulation under local periarticular anesthesia—Part 1: Clinical perspective and pilot study proposal. *JMPT* 7(4):211, 1984

Dr. Wood discusses the posterior primary neural rami, that this neural group supplies the back structures, and that reaction to this rami can extend to include the anterior primary neural rami.

6. Pressman AH, Nickles SL: Neurophysiological and nutritional consideration of pain control. *JMPT* 7(4):219, 1984

This article discusses pain and tissue reaction being a protective mechanism for spinal joints.

7. Dishman R: Review of the literature supporting a scientific basis for the chiropractic subluxation complex. *JMPT* 8(3):163, 1985

The spinal lesion (subluxation) and its relationship to nervous impulses is investigated.

8. Wood L: Acute locked facet syndrome and its treatment by manipulation under local periarticular anesthesia—Part 1: Clinical perspective and pilot study proposal. *JMPT* 7(4):211, 1984

Wood indicates how paraspinal muscle contraction is used by the body as a spinal protective mechanism.

9. Gracovitsky S, Farfan H: The optimum spine. *Spine* 11(6):543, 1986

This article discusses the protective spinal mechanism and the procedures the authors used to determine this action. They have called this action a feedback mechanism. This article is exceptional.

10. Finneson B: *Low Back Pain*, 2nd ed. Philadelphia, JB Lippincott, 1981;p.20

Dr. Finneson indicates that the posterior primary rami of the spinal nerve roots supply sensory fibers to the skin, muscle, fascia, ligaments, and posterior arthrodial joints.

3. CORRELATION BETWEEN PAIN AREA, SPINAL NERVE, AND LESION

Because pain caused by spinal lesions is subjective, the linking of the pain syndrome via the nerve to that area and the spinal level of the lesion is essential in a good orthopedic work-up. The objective findings such as muscle spasm, limited motion, examination findings, x-ray finding, etc., should also be listed because they help to establish the correlation between the pain and the lesion.

When a low back/leg pain case must be adjudicated, it is essential that the doctor follow certain guidelines as set forth in the *AMA Guides to the Evaluation of Permanent Impairment*, 3rd edition. These guidelines are listed on page 66, "Pain," at the top of the second column. They are the following.

A. How the pain interferes with the individual's performance of the activities of daily living; (this of course would be found in the chiropractor's records).
B. To what extent the pain follows the defined anatomical pathways of the root (dermatome), plexus, or peripheral nerve.
C. To what extent the description of the pain indicates that it is caused by the peripheral spinal nerve impairment; how it corresponds to other kinds of disturbances of the involved nerve or nerve root.

The following information, in compliance with these guidelines, identifies the pain syndrome area, the nerve or nerve group involved, and the spinal segments related to that nerve or nerve group, followed by the references that relate specifically to each syndrome area. This information has been given in various sections of this manual, but when shown together they may be better understood by third parties.

A. ***Paraspinal pain syndrome area:*** low back region, unilateral or bilateral, excluding area over the lumbosacral joint
   Spinal level: 9th thoracic to 12th thoracic spinal levels

1. Hamilton WJ: *Textbook of Human Anatomy*, 2nd ed. St. Louis, CV Mosby Co, 1976;p.665
2. Thomas JE: Classification of low back/leg pain—Part 2. *FCA Journal* November–December:18, 1985
3. Thomas JE: Paraspinal pain syndrome—Part 1. *FCA Journal* September–October:27, 1986

B. ***Lumbar pain syndrome area:*** an area over only the 5th lumbar, lumbosacral joint, or both
   Spinal level: 4th and 5th spinal levels

   1. Gray H: *Gray's Anatomy,* 30th ed. Philadelphia, Lea & Febiger, 1984;p.1198
      Nerve supply to deep muscles of the back.
   2. Thomas JE: Classification of low back/leg pain syndromes—Part 2. *FCA Journal* November–December: 18, 1985
   3. Thomas JE: Lumbar pain syndrome—Part 3. *FCA Journal* March–April:52, 1987

C. ***Gluteal pain syndrome area:*** an area approximately the size of a baseball, and located above and lateral to the ischial tuberosity
   Spinal level: 1st, 2nd, and 3rd lumbar spinal levels

   1. Hamilton WJ: *Textbook of Human Anatomy,* 2nd ed. St. Louis, CV Mosby Co, 1976;p.638
      Dorsal primary rami of the 1st, 2nd, and 3rd lumbar nerves to the gluteal region.
   2. Netter F: *Atlas of Human Anatomy,* 2nd ed. Summit NJ, CIBA Pharmaceuticals, 1989;Plate 513
      Superior cluneal nerves to the gluteal region.
   3. Thomas JE: Classification of low back/leg pain syndromes—Part 2. *FCA Journal* November–December: 18, 1985
   4. Thomas JE: Gluteal pain syndrome—Part 5. *FCA Journal* July–August:50, 1987

D. ***Thomas pain syndrome area:*** a small triangle above the trochanter, and a second area extending behind the small area mentioned, fanning out over the posterior lateral gluteus
   Spinal level: 12th thoracic and 1st lumbar spinal levels

   1. Gray H: *Gray's Anatomy,* 30th ed. Philadelphia, Lea & Febiger, 1984;p.1223
      An excellent view is shown of the 12th thoracic and iliohypogastric nerves.
   2. Thomas JE: Classification of low back/leg pain syndromes—Part 2. *FCA Journal* November–December: 18, 1985
   3. Thomas JE: Gluteal pain syndrome—Part 4. *FCA Journal* May–June:34, 1987

E. ***Inguinal pain syndrome area:*** found over the lower abdomen and groin area, may extend slightly into the upper inner thigh unilaterally or bilaterally
   Spinal level: 12th thoracic and 1st lumbar spinal levels.

   1. Gray H: *Gray's Anatomy,* 30th ed. Philadelphia, Lea & Febiger, 1984;p.1224
      A view is shown of the 12th thoracic and iliohypogastric nerves supplying the lower anterior abdominal and groin area.
   2. Thomas JE: Classification of low back/leg pain syndromes—Part 2. *FCA Journal* November–December: 18, 1985
   3. Thomas JE: Inguinal pain syndrome—Part 2. *FCA Journal* November–December:32, 1986

F. ***Anterior femoral pain syndrome area:*** Anterior area of the upper leg to knee
   Spinal level: 2nd, 3rd, and 4th lumbar spinal levels

   1. Gray H: *Gray's Anatomy,* 30th ed. Philadelphia, Lea & Febiger, 1984;p.1229
      These views show the principal area of pain and the nerve distribution.
   2. Hamilton WJ: *Textbook of Human Anatomy,* 2nd ed. St. Louis, CV Mosby Co, 1976;p.659
   3. Thomas JE: Classification of low back/leg pain syndromes—Part 2. *FCA Journal* November–December: 18, 1985
   4. Thomas JE: Anterior femoral pain syndrome. *FCA Journal* September–October:48, 1987

G. ***Lateral femoral pain syndrome area:*** lateral area of the upper leg to knee
   Spinal level: 2nd and 3rd lumbar spinal level.

   1. Gray H: *Gray's Anatomy,* 30th ed. Philadelphia, Lea & Febiger, 1984;p.1229
      The area of distribution for the lateral femoral cutaneous nerve is discussed.
   2. Thomas JE: Classification of low back/leg pain syndromes—Part 2. *FCA Journal* November–December: 18, 1985
   3. Thomas JE: Lateral femoral pain syndrome—Part #7. *FCA Journal* November–December:58, 1987

H. ***Posterior femoral pain syndrome:*** Posterior area of upper leg to knee
   Spinal level: 4th and 5th lumbar spinal level
   (Because this nerve overlays the great sciatic nerve it requires great care in its differential diagnosis.)

   1. Gray H: *Gray's Anatomy,* 30th ed. Philadelphia, Lea & Febiger, 1984;p.1236
      The area of distribution is shown for the posterior femoral nerve.
   2. Netter F: *Atlas of Human Anatomy,* 2nd ed. Summit NJ, CIBA Pharmaceuticals, 1989;Plate 508
   3. Thomas JE: Classification of low back/leg pain syndromes—Part 2. *FCA Journal* November–December: 18, 1985

4. Thomas JE: Posterior femoral pain syndrome—Part 8. *FCA Journal* January–February:56, 1988

4. GENERAL REFERENCES

A few general references are certainly in order and the information can help the physician's relationship with third parties by providing information that may be required as to case management.

1. Hoppenfeld S: *Orthopedic Neurology.* Philadelphia, JB Lippincott, 1977;p.98
   The 12th thoracic vertebra is the most common site of injuries causing paraplegia.
2. Brantingham JW: A survey of literature regarding the behavior, pathology, ideologies and nomenclature of the chiropractic lesion. *Journal of Chiropractic* 22(8):65, 1985
   He discusses how a true subluxation may cause restricted intervertebral motion causing joint pathology with resulting pain.
3. Farfan HF: The use of mechanical etiology to determine the efficacy of active intervention in single joint lumbar intervertebral joint problems. *Spine* 10(4):350, 1985
   This report discusses anatomical variations, and (on pg. 353) joint subluxation to traumatic arthritis and its quiescent phase.
4. Kikuche S, Hasue M, Nishiyama K: Anatomical and clinical studies of radicular symptoms. *Spine* 9(1):23, 1984
   Anatomical variations with radicular syndrome abnormalities are presented.
5. Mayer T, Gatchel R, Kishino N: Objective assessments of spine function following industrial injury. *JMPT* 10(6):482, 1985
   This is a discussion on the number one cause of disability under the age of 45, and the third cause of disability over age 45, related to low back and leg pain.
6. Douglas C, Mooney V, Crame P: Spinal pain rehabilitation: Inpatient and outpatient treatment results and development of predictors for outcome. *Spine* 9(1):91, 1984
   Pathology not predictive of treatment outcome for low back/leg pain cases is discussed.
7. Kirkaldy-Willis WH: *A Scientific Approach: Managing Low Back Pain,* 2nd ed. New York, Churchill Livingstone, 1988;p.93
   The clinical significance of spinal manipulation is presented.
8. Finneson B: *Low Back Pain,* 2nd ed. Philadelphia, JB Lippincott, 1981;p.246
   Present low back examination is unsophisticated, with a poor understanding of the pathogenesis of back pain.
9. White A, McBride M, Wiltse L: The management of patients with back pain and ideopathic vertebral sclerosis. *Spine* 11(6):607, 1986
   This is a discussion of back pain-vertebral sclerosis treatment—after a 6-month and a 2-year follow up.
10. Phillips R, Frymoyer J, Pherson B: Low back pain: A radiographic enigma. *JMPT* 9(3):183, 1986
    X-rays not valid for predicting low back pain.
11. Mayer T, Gatchel R, Kishino N: Objective assessments of spine function following industrial injury. *JMPT* 10(6):482, 1985
    The range-of-motion studies technique is often invalid and misleading.
12. Rocolle A, Bendist M: Surgical findings and results of surgery after failure of chemonucleolysis. *Spine* 10(9):812, 1985
    Failed surgery for low back cases is discussed and indicated as 31%, or more.
13. Higuchi H, Kazuhird A: Effects of hydrocortisone on the vertebral cartilage plate in mice. *Spine* 10(4):297, 1985
    Hydrocortisone causes intervertebral disc and cartilage plate degeneration.
14. Peyster R, Teplick G, Haskin M: Computed tomography of lumbosacral conjointed nerve root anomalies. *Spine* 10(4):331, 1985
    False positive reading with computed tomography is discussed.
15. Morris J, Chafetz N, Baumrind S: Stereophotogrammetry of the lumbar spine. *Spine* 10(4):368, 1985
    Spinal fusion. 30–40% have persistent or recurrent pain.
16. Lincoln F, Manucher J: Cost effectiveness of chemonucleolysis versus laminectomy in the treatment of herniated nucleus pulposus. *Spine* 10(4):363, 1985
    Average cost of chemonucleolysis is $4,163; laminectomy is $6,124.
17. State of Florida, Department of Labor and Employment Security, Division of Workers' Compensation: Part 2—analysis. *1985 Workers' Compensation Injuries.* Tallahasse, State of Florida, Department of Labor and Employment Security, 1985,p.6
    Spinal injuries 35–37% (1982), 34.5% (1983), of all lost time injuries. Average number of days lost was 117.5 (1982), 69 (1983); the average cost per case was $6,412 (1982), $5,190 (1983). Spinal and trunk injuries in 1985 averaged 54 lost days with an average cost of $6,141.
18. Zohn D, Mennell J: *Diagnosis and Physical Treatment, Musculoskeletal Pain,* 1st ed. Boston, Little, Brown & Co. 1976;p.9
    Spinal joint disfunction: Muscle spasm and atrophy are secondary conditions; these may become primary, causing symptoms even after the primary lesion is eradicated.
19. Hoppenfeld S: *Orthopedic Neurology.* Philadelphia, JB Lippincott, 1977;p.67
    Nerve roots carry elements of adjacent nerve roots.
20. Triano J, Luttges M: Myoelectric paraspinal response to spinal loads: Potential for monitoring low back pain. *JMPT* 8(3):137, 1985
21. Waddell G: A new clinical model for the treatment of low back pain. *Spine* 12(7):632, 1987

Information found during this research paper is as follows:

- Bed rest following pain medication appears to be based on a doubtful rationale, with little evidence of a lasting benefit.
- Studies show that controlled exercise aids in restoring function, return to work, and actually reduces pain. Their clinical studies confirm the value of active rehabilitation in practice. Eight controlled studies, and two reviews, show little relationship between clinical symptoms and radiologic changes of degeneration.
- The researchers found that acute cases are more often generally proportionate to the physical findings, that chronic cases appear to be increasingly disassociated from their original physical bases, and that little objective evidence may be present. They indicate that pain clinics are filled with patients who have undergone back surgery.
- One conclusion stated that conventional medical treatment has failed and that the role, then, of medicine must be critically examined. The studies remarked that we must change our entire approach to low back disorders.
- One observation suggested that patients be allowed to draw their own pain areas on figures provided for them. This is not a function that the patient should undertake, because he or she is likely not sufficiently familiar—if at all—with topographical anatomy. When questioned, the patient often extends, in the drawings, beyond the true pain areas suffered.

This article should be read by all doctors who treat low back pain cases and those cases with associated leg pain. Much of the above information is of added interest because the findings confirm the author's own conclusions regarding:

1. acute, reactive spinal segments
2. chronic, (secondary) nonreactive spinal segments and their related pain syndromes

22. Meade T, Dryer S, Browne W: Low back pain of mechanical origin: Randomised comparison of chiropractic and hospital outpatient treatment. *BMJ* 300:431, 1990

    This research program has compared chiropractic and hospital outpatient treatment for managing low back pain of mechanical origin. It has shown that chiropractic treatment is more effective than outpatient hospital management.

23. Members of the Quebec task force for low back leg pain: Treatment of activity-related spinal disorders. *Spine* 12(7s):s22, 1987.

Many more references could be given, but these are the most important in that they offer the treating physician an awareness of the literature that is available related to spinal lesions and their ramifications.

Appendix B

Recommended Information, Graphs, and Forms for Third Parties

The following information is designed to inform and help third parties to understand spinal lesions that cause low back, pelvic, and leg pain. There are two basic types of spinal lesions that do so.

The first type is the gross pathological lesion that can be demonstrated by x-ray, CAT scan, and MRI. Examples of these lesions are spinal birth defects such as lumbarization, sacralization, hemivertebra, tropism, etc.; hereditary spinal lesions such as achondroplasia, Paget's disease, Wilson's disease, juvenile scoliosis, etc; acquired bone disease due to hypervitaminosis, various forms of cancer, thyroid pathologies causing bone changes; almost all forms of arthropathies; arthritis, gout, tuberculosis, degenerative disc disease, hypermobile joints, hypomobile joints, poker spine, etc.; and additionally, the variety of fractures that can be caused by traumatic injury. Disc lesions causing direct nerve pressure and stenosis due to the closure of the intervertebral foramen fall somewhere between gross pathology and the nongross lesion. Occasionally, they can also be determined by present-day diagnostic equipment.

Fortunately for the patient the above-mentioned categories of lesions are not the primary cause of low back, pelvic, and leg pain—a lesion that is elusive to modern equipment and requires a viable orthopedic examination for its determination. This generic lesion is called a subluxation/disrelation, or subluxation.

Gross pathology of the spine causing pain is not difficult to understand, nor is it too difficult to diagnose in most cases. Pain caused by spinal lesions that cannot be seen or detected with present-day diagnostic equipment must, however, be found by connecting the area of pain to the nerve supplying that body area, thus leading to the root level of that nerve. The precise spinal segmental examination can then detect the injured or reactive spinal segment, which may be at the spinal level of the main nerve root, or other spinal levels with associated root fibers, or may be related to the spinal protective mechanism activated because of the spinal trauma.

All spinal pathological conditions including injury can cause back pain and pain away from the spine. This is due to injury or reaction from either or both the anterior and posterior primary neural rami.

Back and radicular pain is not a constant symptom arising from constitutional disease of bone, birth defects, congenital diseases, developmental diseases, or even many old spinal injuries. A patient can have a severe scoliosis, old traumatic spinal joint injuries, or osteoarthritis, even old compression fractures, and be unaware of their existence until a new injury occurs that is superimposed upon the older arthopathies. The new injury causes local tissue reaction that can further aggravate the older, nonreactive, preexisting joint lesion.

There are, of course, exceptions, such as spinal tumors, and so on, and the chiropractor is always on the alert for these conditions.

The basic and most frequent cause of pain resulting from spinal injury, existing with or without the presence of a gross pathological condition, is the subluxation. It is produced by a spinal joint injury, less than a dislocation, and may also be a sequel from spinal arthropathies.[1]

Pain from spinal lesions causes eight major pain syndromes that are found in low back/leg pain cases.[2] The number of these pain syndromes present in any case depends upon the severity of the lesion, nerves involved, and number of spinal levels reactive.

Recent information regarding this lesion provides ample updated versions related to its extent. H. F. Farfan indicates that torsion loads (injury) may cause forced axial lesions due to rotation and lateral flexion. He discusses joint failure and its pain-causing mechanism. He states that torsion injuries (joint subluxation) may develop into traumatic arthritis.[3] S. Hoppenfeld indicates that, due to the structure of the 12th thoracic, it is highly susceptible to injury and is a major cause of paraplegia.[4] J. Wood has written that muscle spasm acts as a protective spinal mechanism, and that mechanical locking by a subluxation causes muscle spasm.[5] J. W. Brantingham discusses restricted intervertebral motion as a cause of pain and joint pathology.[6] H. A. Hadley proved the existence of the subluxation lesion by cadavers with associated nerve pathology.[7] A. B. Good also indicated that joint blocking was a cause of pain and muscle contraction at the spine.[8] R. Dishman discussed the biochemical changes due to lack of movement, and stated that fibrosis with scar tissue is the result.[9] S. M. Forman indicated that ossification of the posterior longitudinal ligament could be a cause of stenosis.[10] The pathoanatomy and pathophysiology of nerve root compression was written by Rydevik, Brown, and Lundborg, and they also indicated how compression of a dorsal nerve root ganglion produced repetitive firing, causing pain.[11] A. H. Pressman also coupled the subluxation lesion with neural impulses.[12] There are many more references, but these should give a good sample of current thought and findings related to the spinal lesion.

As the above information and the location of the lesion is considered, it must be apparent that this lesion is capable of causing additional pathology and reaction to tissues not found immediately at its site, that it can exist within a pathological condition, and can become pathological within its own right to the point of additional joint or soft tissue destruction. This is the definition of this nongross spinal lesion.

A subluxation/disrelation lesion is an abnormal relationship at the joint between two bony structures, that is present during motion and the transitional stage, and that continues to exist in a static position. This disrelationship is a pathological entity with tissue reaction as its sequel. This pathological entity can be disrelated both anatomically, physiologically, or both.[13]

Types of Subluxations

1. **Primary.** *A subluxation/disrelation spinal joint injury without previous injury or pathology to that spinal level.*
2. **Secondary.** *A subluxation/disrelation injury superimposed upon a previous spinal joint injury or existing spinal joint pathology or constitutional disease of bone.*

Subclassifications of a Subluxation/Disrelation Lesion

1. Trophic lesions
2. Vascular lesion
3. Neural lesions
4. Facet lesions
5. Disc lesions
6. Other soft-tissue lesions
7. Bone lesions (injury, disease, congenital)
8. Hypomobility of vertebral segments
9. Hypermobility of vertebral segments
10. Any combination of the above

Symptoms of a Subluxation

1. Protective muscle splinting
2. Low back pain, posterior primary rami reaction, due to joint injury and splinting
3. Known body areas of pain due to anterior and posterior primary nerve root injury, reaction, or both
4. Paresthesia may occur in the more serious nerve injuries
5. Acute traumatic arthritis, all contributing to
6. Disability due to pain, muscle contraction, and tissue changes of the spinal motor unit

Pain Syndromes Caused by a Subluxation/Disrelation Injury

1. Paraspinal syndrome
2. Lumbar syndrome
3. Gluteal syndrome
4. Thomas syndrome
5. Inguinal syndrome
6. Anterior femoral syndrome
7. Lateral femoral syndrome
8. Posterior femoral syndrome
9. Sciatic syndrome: This syndrome is usually due to disc lesion and occurs in less than one half of 1% of low back/leg pain cases.

Nerve Divisions and Major Nerves That May Be Involved in a Subluxation/Disrelation Injury

1. Dorsal primary rami
2. Anterior primary rami
3. Superior cluneal nerves
4. 12th thoracic nerve
5. Iliohypogastric nerve
6. Ilioinguinal nerve
7. 1st lumbar nerve
8. Genitofemoral nerve
9. Femoral nerve
10. Lateral femoral cutaneous nerve
11. Posterior femoral cutaneous nerve
12. Sciatic nerve

The above is only a portion of the knowledge related to this nongross spinal lesion.

A question that must be answered is this: Pain is a subjective symptom. What are its objective indications that can be found and recorded?

Although pain is a subjective symptom, its presence must have some foundation. By indicating the pain syndrome area, the patient's pain within that area, the nerve supplying that body area, the spinal level from which that nerve arises, and its lesion, the anatomical circle for pain is completed.

When the specific injury is described, the result of the forces caused by that injury should be included, such as hyperflexion, hyperextension, abnormal lateral flexion, torque, whiplash, stretch, compression, etc. The type of force such as blows, crushing, pushing, pulling, lifting, falling, etc., should also be indicated. These forces cause the lesion that produces pain and injury to the nerve or nerves, and results in an activated syndrome area, thus establishing the foundation for the total injury complex.

The objective findings are the building blocks that are required to further substantiate the presence of a spinal lesion that causes pain. For some reason, the recording of these symptoms is often overlooked by physicians. Test findings, positive or negative, found during the orthopedic examination are, of course, one form of objective finding. Painful fibrotic nodules at muscle attachments particularly along the iliac crests are also objective findings, but of most importance is the contraction of paraspinal muscles. These contracted muscles can be palpated, are usually painful during palpation, and often can be seen when standing motion studies are conducted. Muscle contraction can generally be found by palpation 2 to 3 inches lateral to the spinous process, and is often quite visible when observing the patient from the back when he or she bends forward in a flexed position. If the patient is unable to stand erect due to muscle contraction, the muscles responsible for this status can be palpated and should be listed. Any minor restricted motion should be indicated; gross restricted movement is a basis for impairment ratings. It was indicated earlier in this manual, that anterior posterior and lateral x-rays are the minimum number of films that should be taken. Additionally, lateral flexion studies often show differences in paraspinal muscle density, as well as vertebral segments that are locked-in and are restricted in lateral flexion due to deep muscle contraction. Anterior flexion and extension studies in some cases may be required, especially at the cervical region, following an auto injury, to determine the stability of the spinal joint. All gross pathology that has even a remote connection to the injured joint(s) should be noted, particularly if it is found within the area of the lumbosacral plexus up to and including the 10th thoracic vertebra. This gross pathology constitutes secondary spinal lesions that play a part in the overall picture, although they may have been dormant or painfree, prior to the injury.

With this information properly indicated, the chiropractor establishes a complete profile from *causation* to end results, *pain*.

One important diagnostic error that is frequently seen on physician's reports is the use of the terms low back strain or sprain.

Dorland's *Illustrated Medical Dictionary* defines *strain* as, *over exercise, and/or overstretching some part of the musculature.*

(When rested for a few days, *a patient with this problem* may return to normal.) Any treatment given is certainly minimal. This diagnosis is never indicated in the presence of a spinal joint lesion.

Dorland's defines *sprain* as *the wrenching of a joint with partial rupture or other injury to its attachments, and without luxation of bone. The signs of a sprain are rapid swelling, heat, and disablement of the joint. The pain is usually great, and is much increased by movement.*

Spinal joints are, of course, subject to sprain, as are most joints of the body. A traumatic or sudden injury must have occurred prior to the pain and disability. Most important with spinal joint sprain, however, is the added injury caused to the tissues that lie within the intervertebral foramen, particularly members of the nervous system.

It is mandatory that the chiropractor indicate these more important additional lesions that occur concurrently with spinal joint sprain, and record the associated subjective and objective symptoms.

A spinal joint sprain always produces injury to inferforamenal tissues, including members of the neural system.

Time is important to the chiropractor, whether treating 100 patients per day, or 25. The method used to inform third parties requires part of that time, and in some cases it is considerable. The more time spent writing narrative reports, the less time available to treat patients who needs attention. The status of reporting has increased over the past few years, and there is no indication that it will be reduced over the next decade; in fact, every indicator points to increases in required paperwork.

The author has endeavored to create forms that can eliminate a large percentage of the previous narrative work required and still give the important, necessary information.

This chapter provides forms for each pain syndrome area. If, for an example, a patient is found to have pain within the areas of both the paraspinal pain syndrome and the anterior femoral pain syndrome, each form, with the patient's name and insurance number, can be sent. Should the patient's pain extend outside the pain syndrome area, it can be added with pen or pencil. If the pain area suffered by the patient is localized in a smaller area within the pain syndrome, it can be shown using a red pen. This reduces the time spent on a lengthy narrative report giving the perimeters of the patient's pain and, equally important, when a progress report is required, the changes in the pain area can be shown on the additional forms submitted. Note Forms 101 through 108.

APPENDIX B: RECOMMENDED INFORMATION, GRAPHS, AND FORMS

Doctor's Name
Address

Pat. Name: _____ Ins. # _____

The following graph shows the spine, the spinal vertebral layer, and the nerve or nerves to the area of pain suffered by this patient. The pain may or may not cover the entire area shown in this chart. These pain syndrome areas are bilateral, but many patients suffer from pain only on one side.

Paraspinal Pain Syndrome (Posterior Primary Rami)

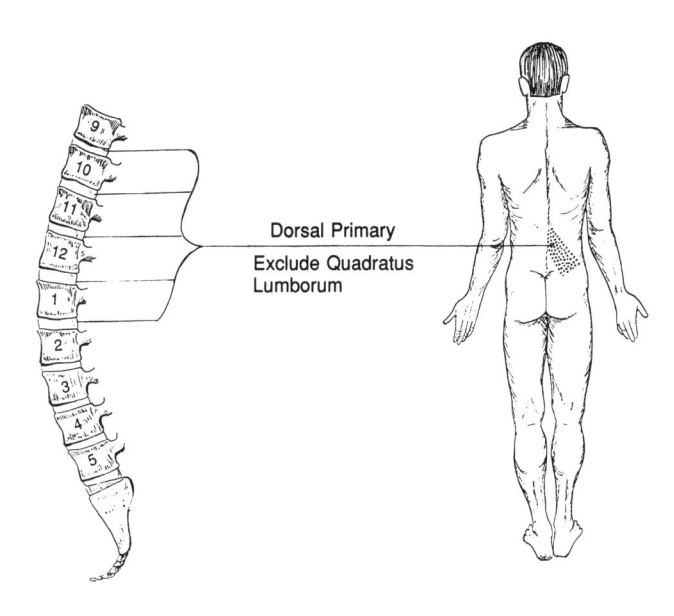

Dorsal Primary

Exclude Quadratus Lumborum

This pain area, involving one or both sides of the body, is found in 60% of low back/leg pain cases. The pain in this region is complex and caused by spinal joint injury or pathology to those spinal joints. Soft tissue injury activates the spinal nerves causing muscle contraction for protection. This muscle activity associated with the joint injury produces pain.

It is essential that the patient stop all forms of exercise, house or yard work, etc., until the pain abates. Treatment should be continued until the injured spinal joint is no longer sensitive to pressure.

(c) J.E. THOMAS, D.C. F.A.C.O. 1984   form 101

Doctor's Name
Address

Pat. Name: _   Ins. # _ _ _ _ _ _ _ _ _ _ _ _

The following graph shows the spine, the spinal vertebral level, and the nerve or nerves to the area of pain suffered by this patient. The pain may or may not cover the entire area shown in this chart. These pain syndrome areas are bilateral, but many patients suffer from pain only on one side.

Lumbar Pain Syndrome (Posterior Primary Rami)

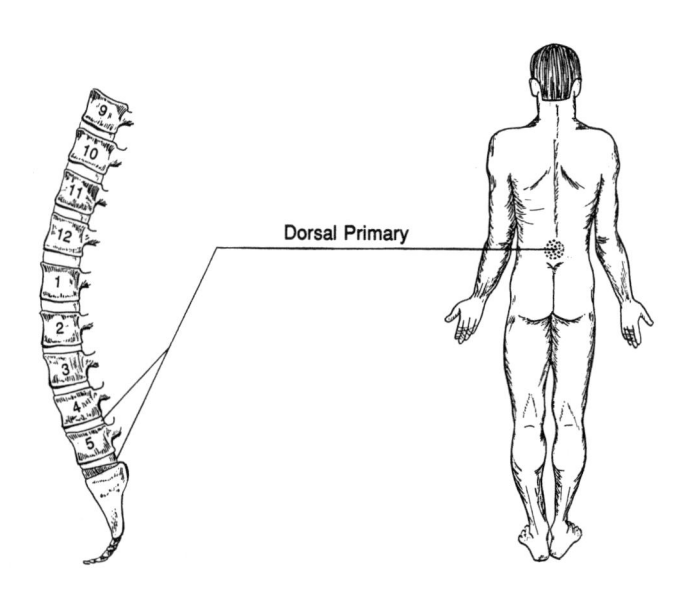

Dorsal Primary

This pain area, shown in this drawing, is found when injury occurs to the 4th or 5th lumbar spinal segments. Most frequently it is the 5th lumbar or lumbosacral joint. Bending and twisting appear to be the positions most frequently noted preceding the injury to this spinal area. Pain may be immediate or delayed for some period of time.

All activities should be stopped as long as the pain is present. Treatment should be continued until all pain is gone, when pressure is applied to the reactive joint.

(c) J.E. THOMAS, D.C. F.A.C.O. 1984   form 102

APPENDIX B: RECOMMENDED INFORMATION, GRAPHS, AND FORMS   129

Doctor's Name
Address

Pat. Name: _   Ins. # _ _ _ _ _ _ _ _ _ _ _ _ _ _

The following graph shows the spine, the spinal vertebral level, and the nerve or nerves to the area of pain suffered by this patient. The pain may or may not cover the entire area shown in this chart. These pain syndrome areas are bilateral, but many patients suffer from pain only on one side.

Inguinal Pain Syndrome (Anterior Primary Rami)

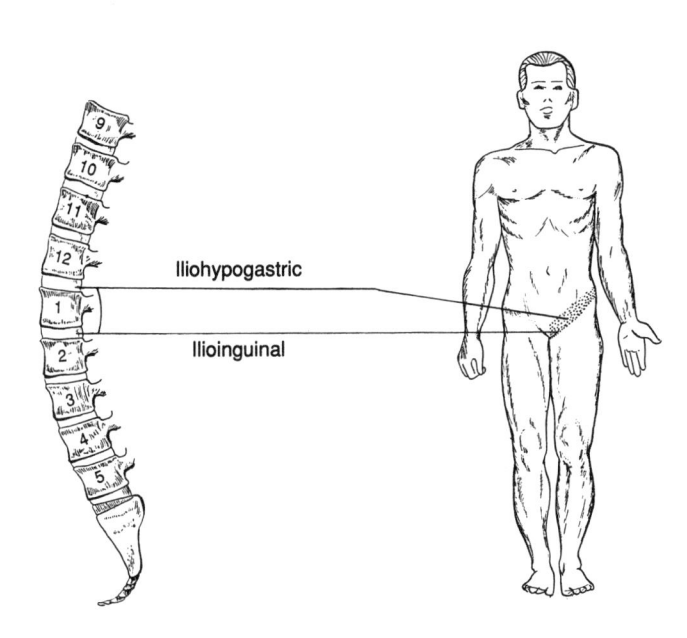

Iliohypogastric

Ilioinguinal

This pain area can involve one or two nerves. It is caused by spinal joint injury with associated nerve root injury.

A note of interest: This syndrome for many years has been considered prevalent in females and possibly connected to gynecological problems. Since more recent research has shown it occurs twice as frequently to males, that idea no longer has any foundation.

Stop all exercise and reduce other activity until joint examination proves total reduction of joint pain.

(c) J.E. THOMAS, D.C. F.A.C.O. 1984   form 103

Doctor's Name
Address

Pat. Name: _   Ins. # _ _ _ _ _ _ _ _ _ _ _ _

The following graph shows the spine, the spinal vertebral level, and the nerve or nerves to the area of pain suffered by this patient. The pain may or may not cover the entire area shown in this chart. These pain syndrome areas are bilateral, but many patients suffer from pain only on one side.

Thomas Pain Syndrome (Anterior Primary Rami)

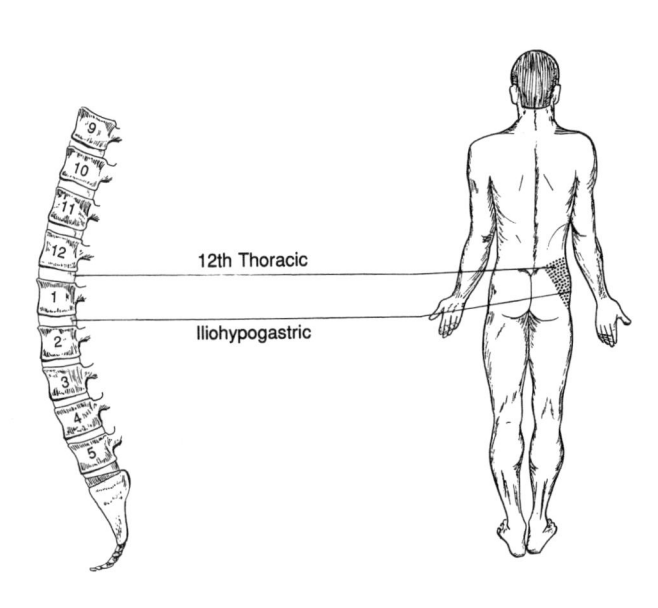

- 12th Thoracic
- Iliohypogastric

This pain area is complex, it may involve one or two joints. Each joint contains a nerve root that when injured causes pain that overlays the hip region.

All exercise and walking must be restricted until pain in this area is stopped. Treatment should continue until the injured joints are pain free on examination.

(c) J.E. THOMAS, D.C. F.A.C.O. 1984   form 104

Doctor's Name
Address

Pat. Name: _   Ins. # _ _ _ _ _ _ _ _ _ _ _ _

The following graph shows the spine, the spinal vertebral level, and the nerve or nerves to the area of pain suffered by this patient. The pain may or may not cover the entire area shown in this chart. These pain syndrome areas are bilateral, but many patients suffer from pain only on one side.

Gluteal Pain Syndrome (Posterior Primary Rami)

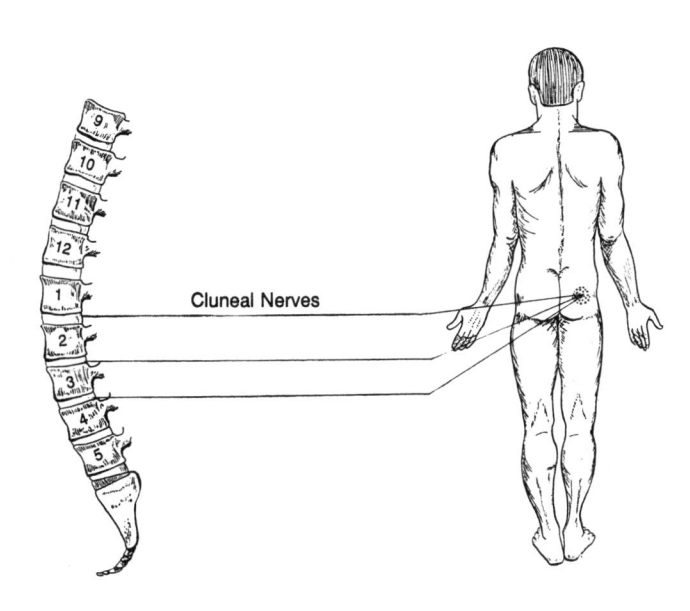

Cluneal Nerves

This pain area, found in the pelvic region, is caused by spinal joint injury that causes nerve reaction. The nerve root irritation causes the pain to this region.

All exercise and activities, including bending and twisting, should be stopped until the pain is gone or under control. Treatment should continue until the spinal joint is no longer sensitive to pressure.

(c) J.E. THOMAS, D.C. F.A.C.O. 1984   form 105

132 CHIROPRACTIC MANUAL OF LOW BACK AND LEG PAIN

Doctor's Name
Address

Pat. Name: _ _ _ _ _ _ _ _ _ _ _ _ _ _ _ _ _ _ _   Ins. # _ _ _ _ _ _ _ _ _ _ _

The following graph shows the spine, the spinal vertebral level, and the nerve or nerves to the area of pain suffered by this patient. The pain may or may not cover the entire area shown in this chart. These pain syndrome areas are bilateral, but many patients suffer from pain only on one side.

Anterior Femoral Pain Syndrome (Anterior Primary Rami)

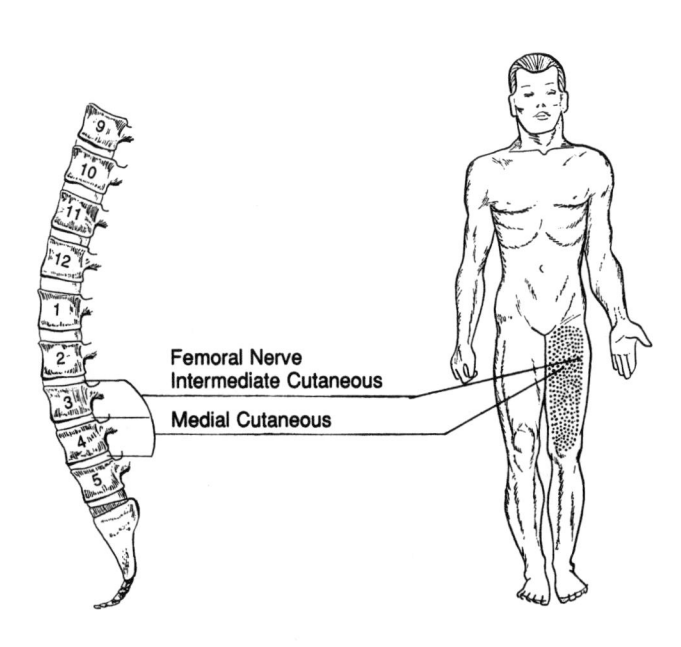

Femoral Nerve
Intermediate Cutaneous
Medial Cutaneous

This pain area is most common as shown on the drawing. Some cases will have knee pain and those cases with greater injury may have pain down the inside of the lower leg to the toe. Injury to the spinal joints, resulting in neural and soft tissue reaction are the cause of this pain area.

Activities must be restricted until the leg pain is stopped. Treatment should continue until the injured joints and nerve roots can be examined free from pain.

(c) J.E. THOMAS, D.C. F.A.C.O. 1984 form 106

APPENDIX B: RECOMMENDED INFORMATION, GRAPHS, AND FORMS   133

Doctor's Name
Address

Pat. Name: _   Ins. # _ _ _ _ _ _ _ _ _ _ _ _

The following graph shows the spine, the spinal vertebral level, and the nerve or nerves to the area of pain suffered by this patient. The pain may or may not cover the entire area shown in this chart. These pain syndrome areas are bilateral, but many patients suffer from pain only on one side.

Lateral Femoral Pain Syndrome (Anterior Primary Rami)

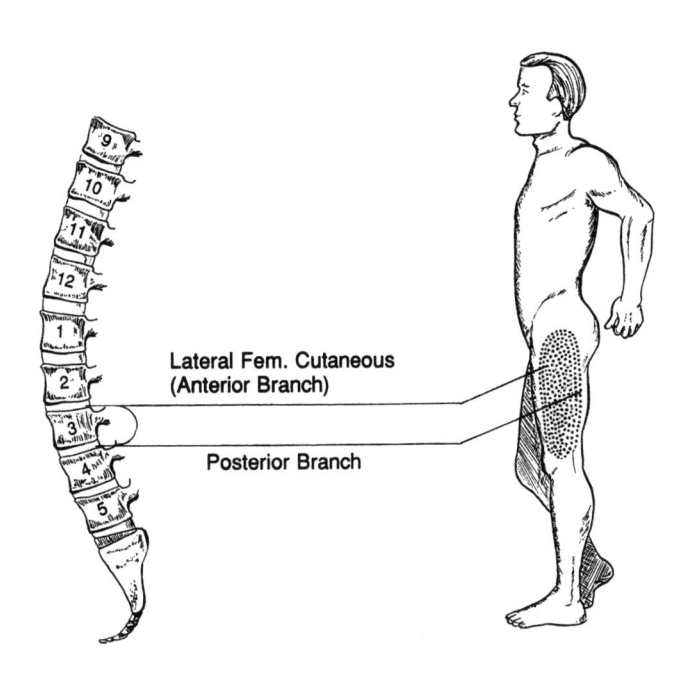

Lateral Fem. Cutaneous (Anterior Branch)
Posterior Branch

This pain syndrome is caused by injury to spinal joints that affect the lateral femoral cutaneous nerve, and is brought about by bending and lifting. It appears to affect men and women on an equal basis.

All activities should be restricted while pain is present. Treatment should continue until joint pain on pressure is abated.

(c) J.E. THOMAS, D.C. F.A.C.O. 1984   form 107

134 CHIROPRACTIC MANUAL OF LOW BACK AND LEG PAIN

Doctor's Name
Address

Pat. Name: _ _ _ _ _ _ _ _ _ _ _ _ _ _ _ _ _ _   Ins. # _ _ _ _ _ _ _ _ _ _ _ _

The following graph shows the spine, the spinal vertebral level, and the nerve or nerves to the area of pain suffered by this patient. The pain may or may not cover the entire area shown in this chart. These pain syndrome areas are bilateral, but many patients suffer from pain only on one side.

Posterior Femoral Pain Syndrome (Anterior Primary Rami)

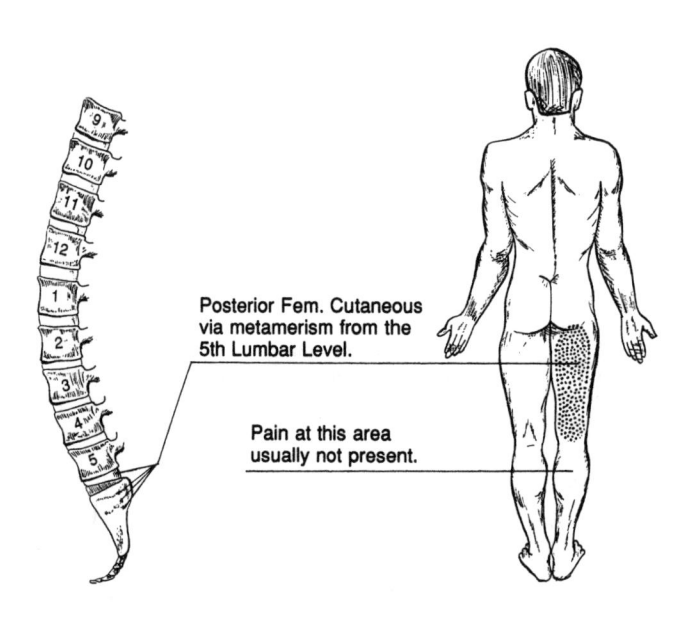

Posterior Fem. Cutaneous via metamerism from the 5th Lumbar Level.

Pain at this area usually not present.

This pain syndrome is highly complex and caused by spinal joint injury at the lowest spinal level. It may, in severe cases, extend below the knee. When pain is present in the low back with this pain syndrome, muscle spasm is usually present and it can be severe.

Total restriction of all activities is necessary to reduce swelling and inflammation around the nerve root, and to aid in the prevention of permanent damage to soft tissue. Treatment should continue until all leg pain is gone, and the injured joint is free from pain on pressure.

(c) J.E. THOMAS, D.C. F.A.C.O. 1984   form 108

REFERENCES FOR FORMS 101 THROUGH 108

Form 101. Paraspinal Pain Syndrome

Gray H: *Gray's Anatomy,* 30th ed. Philadelphia, Lea & Febiger, 1984;pp.466–473

Form 102. Lumbar Pain Syndrome

Gray H: *Gray's Anatomy,* 30th ed. Philadelphia, Lea & Febiger, 1984;pp.1197
Netter F: *Atlas of Human Anatomy,* 2nd ed. Summit NJ, CIBA Pharmaceuticals, 1989;Plate 163

Form 103. Inguinal Pain Syndrome

Gray H: *Gray's Anatomy,* 30th ed. Philadelphia, Lea & Febiger, 1984;p.1227
Netter F: *Atlas of Human Anatomy,* 2nd ed. Summit NJ, CIBA Pharmaceuticals, 1989;Plate 512

Form 104. Thomas Pain Syndrome

Gray H: *Gray's Anatomy,* 30th ed. Philadelphia, Lea & Febiger, 1984;p.1227

Form 105. Gluteal Pain Syndrome

Gray H: *Gray's Anatomy,* 30th ed. Philadelphia, Lea & Febiger, 1984;p.1195
Netter F: *Atlas of Human Anatomy,* 2nd ed. Summit NJ, CIBA Pharmaceuticals, 1989;Plate 513

Form 106. Anterior Femoral Pain Syndrome

Gray H: *Gray's Anatomy,* 30th ed. Philadelphia, Lea & Febiger, 1984;p.1231
Netter F: *Atlas of Human Anatomy,* 2nd ed. Summit NJ, CIBA Pharmaceuticals, 1989;Plate 506

Form 107. Lateral Femoral Pain Syndrome

Gray H: *Gray's Anatomy,* 30th ed. Philadelphia, Lea & Febiger, 1984;p.1229
Netter F: *Atlas of Human Anatomy,* 2nd ed. Summit NJ, CIBA Pharmaceuticals, 1989;Plate 506

Form 108. Posterior Femoral Pain Syndrome

Gray H: *Gray's Anatomy,* 30th ed. Philadelphia, Lea & Febiger, 1984;p.1236
Netter F: *Atlas of Human Anatomy,* 2nd ed. Summit NJ, CIBA Pharmaceuticals, 1989;Plate 508
Hoppenfeld S: *Orthopedic Neurology.* Philadelphia, JB Lippincott, 1977;p.67
Turek S: *Orthopaedics: Principles and Their Application,* 3rd ed. Philadelphia, JB Lippincott, 1959;p.67
Best CH, Taylor NB: *The Physiological Basis of Medical Practice,* 4th ed. Baltimore, Williams & Wilkins, 1945;p.847

Examination forms for low back/pelvic/leg pain are presented, and are designed to give the required information showing both the positive and negative findings as well as the areas of pain suffered by the patient. Blocks can be checked to indicate the pain syndrome suffered by the patient. The pain syndrome forms when attached to the examination forms for a report, reduce considerably the time required for a narrative report. They give an accurate accounting of the patient's condition related to low back, pelvic, and leg pain. Note examination forms 109, 110, and 111.

CERVICAL/UPPER THORACIC EXAMINATION

Dr.'s Name. _____
Address. _____
_____

Dr.'s Ph. No. _____
Date: _____/_____/_____

Patient's name: _____ Ins. # _____

The following examination procedures are completed on all patients suffering from pain syndromes resulting from cervical, and/or upper thoracic pathology or injury. No part of this examination is ever deleted. Findings both negative and positive are recorded and considered for a final determination. Neck, shoulder, arm and/or upper thoracic pain syndromes are present before this examination is started. Failure to follow a precise procedure leads to false findings which can mislead the physician and result in an incorrect diagnosis and treatment.

RANGE OF MOTION:

FLEXION: NEG. _____ POS. _____ PAIN AREA. _____
_____ % LOSS. _____

EXTENSION: NEG. _____ POS. _____ PAIN AREA. _____
_____ % LOSS. _____

RIGHT FLEX: NEG. _____ POS. _____ PAIN AREA. _____
_____ % LOSS. _____

LEFT FLEX: NEG. _____ POS. _____ PAIN AREA. _____
_____ % LOSS. _____

RT. ROTATION: NEG. _____ POS. _____ PAIN AREA. _____
_____ % LOSS. _____

LEFT ROTATION: NEG. _____ POS. _____ PAIN AREA. _____

NECK COMPRESSION TESTS

STRAIGHT DOWN: NEG. _____ POS. _____ PAIN AREA. _____
_____

PRESSURE RIGHT: NEG. _____ POS. _____ PAIN AREA. _____
_____

PRESSURE LEFT: NEG. _____ POS. _____ PAIN AREA. _____
_____

SPECIAL TESTS:

KEMP SIGN: RT. NEG. ___ POS. ___ LEFT. NEG. ___ POS. ___
COMMENT. _____
SHOULDER DEPRESSION TEST: RT. NEG. _____ POS. _____
LEFT. NEG. _____ POS. _____ COMMENT: _____

Additional tests that might be required and/or comments related to the above examination:

_____
_____
_____

PROBE TO CERVICAL AND UPPER THORACIC VERTEBRAE FOR PAIN: CODE: S. sensitive, P. pain, SH, sharp, H. highly reactive to pressure.

	NEG.	S L/R	P L/R	SH L/R	HR L/R		NEG.	S L/R	P L/R	SH L/R	HR L/R
Base of skull:	____	___/___	___/___	___/___	___/___	1st T.	____	___/___	___/___	___/___	___/___
3rd/4th Cerv:	____	___/___	___/___	___/___	___/___	2nd T.	____	___/___	___/___	___/___	___/___
4th/5th Cerv:	____	___/___	___/___	___/___	___/___	3rd T.	____	___/___	___/___	___/___	___/___
5th/6th Cerv:	____	___/___	___/___	___/___	___/___	4th T.	____	___/___	___/___	___/___	___/___
7th Cerv:	____	___/___	___/___	___/___	___/___	5th T.	____	___/___	___/___	___/___	___/___
						6th T.	____	___/___	___/___	___/___	___/___

Vascular changes and signs from cervical pathology when observed will be noted below. Intercostal pain when found during the segmental examination will also be noted in the space below.

X-RAY FINDINGS: _____
_____
_____

CONCLUSIONS: _____
_____
_____

(c) J.E. Thomas D.C. F.A.C.O. 1984

form 109

Dr.'s Name. _____
Address. _____

LOW BACK/LEG PAIN EXAMINATION

Dr.'s Ph. No. _____
Date: ____/____/____

Patient's name: _____ Ins. #. _____

The following examination procedures are completed on all patients suffering from pain syndromes resulting from low back pathology or injury. No part of this examination is ever deleted. Findings both negative and positive are recorded and considered for a final determination. Low back/leg pain syndromes are present before this examination is started. Failure to follow a precise procedure leads to false findings which can mislead the physician and result in an incorrect diagnosis and treatment.

STRAIGHT LEG RAISING TEST:

   R: NEG. _____ POS. _____ PAIN AREA. _____
_____

   L: NEG. _____ POS. _____ PAIN AREA. _____
_____

FABERE:

   R: NEG. _____ POS. _____ PAIN AREA. _____
_____

   L: NEG. _____ POS. _____ PAIN AREA. _____
_____

SOTO HALL

   NEG. _____ POS. _____ LEVEL. _____
_____

LINDERS:

   NEG. _____ POS. _____ LEVEL. _____

SITTING STRAIGHT LEG RAISING: The patient is not allowed to brace himself/herself, while sitting for this test.

   R: NEG. _____ POS. _____ PAIN AREA. _____
_____

   L: NEG. _____ POS. _____ PAIN AREA. _____
_____

OBJECTIVE SYMPTOMS, AND AREA, NOTED DURING THIS EXAMINATION:
_____
_____

CONCLUSION FOR THIS PORTION OF THE EXAMINATION: _____
_____
_____
_____

In order to aid a third party in the anatomical and neurological connection between the injured and/or reactive spinal segments and the pain area, we have enclosed a copy of that pain syndrome, showing the neural connection (with the nerve or nerve group listed), and the spinal level that these nerves or nerve groups arise from. It must also be remembered that fibers from each nerve arise from one or two levels above and below these listed spinal segments via metamerism. note: References are present to aid the third party in the further investigation of these anatomical connections and spinal levels. This information complies with guidelines as set forth on pg 66 of *Guides to the Evaluation of Permanent Impairment*, 3rd ed, published by the AMA.

ENCLOSED is a copy of the pain syndrome area suffered by the patient. This is a permanent part of the patient's record:

PARASPINAL PAIN SYNDROME ☐	THOMAS PAIN SYNDROME ☐	LATERAL FEMORAL PAIN SYNDROME ☐
LUMBAR PAIN SYNDROME ☐	GLUTEAL PAIN SYNDROME ☐	POSTERIOR FEMORAL PAIN SYNDROME ☐
INGUINAL PAIN SYNDROME ☐	ANTERIOR FEM. PAIN SYNDROME ☐	SCIATIC PAIN SYNDROME ☐

(c) J.E. Thomas D.C. F.A.C.O. 1984

form 110

Dr.'s Name. _____
Address. _____
_____

LOW BACK/LEG PAIN EXAMINATION

Dr.'s Ph. No. _____
Date: _____/_____/_____

Patient's name: _____ Ins. # _____

The following portion of the examination, for low back/leg pain, is a spinal segmental examination designed to examine each spinal segment over a precise spinal area that contains elements of the spine, subject to injury or reaction. These injured or reactive elements cause the symptoms of pain and muscle contraction found in low back/leg pain cases. This examination is conducted on all patients with low back, groin, hip, and leg pain that can be associated with spinal lesions. It is also used when periodic progress reports are necessary.

Code: N: negative, S: sensitive, P: painful, SH: sharp, H: highly reactive, RECORD PAIN AREA IF POSITIVE.

SUPRASPINAL LIGAMENT:
   NEG. _____ S. _____ P. _____ HR. _____ SH. _____

(THIS PAIN AREA WOULD ONLY BE FOUND AT THE LUMBOSACRAL JOINT)

THORACIC SEGMENTS:

	NEG.	S L/R	P L/R	SH L/R	HR L/R
10T	____	___/___	___/___	___/___	___/___
11T	____	___/___	___/___	___/___	___/___
12T	____	___/___	___/___	___/___	___/___

X-RAY REPORT: _____
_____
_____

REPORT FROM CAT SCAN AND/OR MRI IF REQUIRED: _____
_____
_____
_____

LUMBAR SEGMENTS:

1L	____	___/___	___/___	___/___	___/___
2L	____	___/___	___/___	___/___	___/___
3L	____	___/___	___/___	___/___	___/___
4L	____	___/___	___/___	___/___	___/___
5L	____	___/___	___/___	___/___	___/___

CONCLUSIONS: _____
_____
_____
_____
_____

This condensed method is best suited for a status report rather than a narrative report, but is effective for a quick review of the case.

CONDENSED STATUS OR PROGRESS REPORT

1. NAME OF PAIN SYNDROME OR SYNDROMES   : _____
2. PRIMARY OR SECONDARY LESION   : _____
3. REACTION RATING FOR SLR TEST AT 5L MOTOR UNIT   : _____
4. REACTION RATING FOR SPINAL SEGMENTAL TEST AT 5TH L   : _____
5. REACTION RATING FOR SPINAL SEGMENTAL TEST AT 12TH T   : _____
6. REACTION RATING FOR OTHER SPINAL SEGMENTS   : _____
7. OBJECTIVE SYMPTOMS RELATED TO THE PAIN AREA   : _____

(c) J.E. Thomas D.C. F.A.C.O. 1984

form 111

For Medicare and other insurance companies requiring frequent, but not narrative reports, Form 112 is specifically designed to answer the major questions asked: this form can be filled out in a few moments.

A Physician's Desk Manual reflects the latest information known, related to the subject written about. Future advances in low back, pelvic, and leg pain should be incorporated periodically to keep the doctor up to date. It is hoped that the first edition of this manual is only the beginning.

MEDICARE/INSURANCE

Dr.'s Name. _____
Address _____
City _____
State _____ Zip _____

Date: _____/_____/_____
Physician's No. _____
Phone No. _____

Patient's Name: _____ MC#/Ins. #. _____

Place an X on the Appropriate Line

AREA OF COMPLAINT: Suboccipital _____ Cerv. Brac: _____ Dorsal: _____
DORSOCOSTAL: _____ Low Back: _____ Pelvis: _____ Legs: _____
PHYSICAL FINDINGS. (SUBJECTIVE): Pain: _____ Ache: _____ Mild: _____
Sharp: _____ Severe: _____ Burning: _____ Other: _____
Paresthesia: _____
(OBJECTIVE): Restricted Motion: Yes _____ No _____
Muscle Contraction: Yes _____ No _____ Contusion: Yes _____ No _____
Redness: Yes _____ No _____ Swelling: Yes _____ No _____
SPINAL LEVEL INJURED AND/OR REACTIVE: Cervical. 1. _____ 2. _____ 3. _____ 4. _____
5. _____ 6. _____ 7. _____ Thoracic. 1. _____ 2. _____ 3. _____ 4. _____ 5. _____ 6. _____ 7. _____
8. _____ 9. _____ 10. _____ 11. _____ 12. _____ Lumbar. 1. _____ 2. _____ 3. _____ 4. _____ 5. _____
LOW BACK, PELVIC, LEG PAIN SYNDROME: Lumbar. _____ Paraspinal. _____
Inguinal. _____ Thomas. _____ Gluteal. _____ Ant. Fem. _____ Lat. Fem. _____
Pos. Fem. _____ . Cervical/Thoracic: _____
PRE-EXISTING PATHOLOGY: Degenerative Joint Disease: Yes _____ No _____
Birth Defects: Yes _____ No _____ Other Gross Pathology: Yes _____ No _____
Estimated Prognosis: Good _____ Fair _____ Poor _____
Permanent Disability: _____ Estimated No. Treatements Per Mo. _____
Required for This Condition. Estimated No. Months _____ for Conntrol or Correction.
Treatment Required to Reduce Severe Pain: Yes _____ No _____
Treatment Required to Prevent Further Joint Injury: Yes _____ No _____
Pathology Noted on X-Ray Findings: _____
_____
Attached and Part of This Record (Subluxation/Disrelation) Description—Will Be Sent upon Request.
Attached and Part of This Record (Pain Syndromes)—Illustration, Graphics—Showing Area of Pain, Nerve Supply and References.
SYNDROME NAME: _____
_____

(THESE GRAPHICS SHOW THE PAIN AREA SUFFERED BY THIS PATIENT.)

(c) 1988 J.E. Thomas D.C. F.A.C.O.

form 112

REFERENCES FOR FORMS 109 THROUGH 112

1. Farfan HF: The use of mechanical etiology to determine the efficacy of active intervention in single joint lumbar intervertebral joint problems. *Spine* 10(4): 350, 1985
2. Thomas JE: Classification of low back/leg pain—Part 2. *FCA Journal* November–December: 18, 1985
3. Farfan HF: The use of mechanical etiology to determine the efficacy of active intervention in single joint lumbar intervertebral joint problems. *Spine* 10(4): 350, 1985
4. Hoppenfeld S: *Orthopedic Neurology*. Philadelphia, JB Lippincott, 1977;p.98
5. Wood L: Acute locked facet syndrome and its treatment by manipulation under local periarticular anesthesia—Part 1: Clinical perspective and pilot study proposal. *JMPT* 7(4):211, 1984
6. Brantingham JW: A survey of literature regarding the behavior, pathology, ideologies and nomenclature of the chiropractic lesion. *Journal of Chiropractic* 22(8):65, 1985
   He discusses how a true subluxation may cause restricted intervertebral motion causing joint pathology with resulting pain.
7. Hadley LA: Intervertebral joint subluxation, bony impingement and foramen encroachment with nerve root changes. *AJR* 26(3):377, 1951
8. Good AB: Spinal joint blocking. *JMPT* 8(1):1, 1985
9. Dishman R: Review of the literature supporting a scientific basis for the chiropractic subluxation complex. *JMPT* 8(3):163, 1985
10. Foreman SM: Ossification of posterior longitudinal ligament a cause of spinal stenosis. *JMPT* 7(1),1984:253
11. Rydevik B, Mark Brown, Goran Lundborg: Pathoanatomy and pathophysiology of nerve root compression. *Spine* 9(1):7, 1984
12. Pressman AH, Nickles SL: Neurophysiological and nutritional consideration of pain control. *JMPT* 7(4): 219, 1984
13. Thomas JE: Classification of low back/leg pain syndromes—Part 4. *FCA Journal* March–April:32, 1986

To aid those physicians who would like to use the various forms found in this manual, examination forms, insurance and medicare forms, pain syndrome forms, "Important Information for Third Parties" references found in Appendix B, and so on, can be copied from the manual on an individual case basis when needed. *Copies cannot be reproduced by any method for private or commercial resale or general distribution.*

Index

Anatomical nerve variation, 17, 19, 58, 62
Antalgic splinting, 10, 15, 53
Anterior femoral pain syndrome, 6, 69
Anterior primary rami, 12, 17

Bed rest, 101
Body regions, 2
   leg region, 6
      perimeter, 3
   pelvic region, 5
      perimeter, 3
   low back region, 4
      perimeter, 3
Bowstring sign, 35
Braggards, 80
Buckling sign, 35

CAT (computer assisted tomography) scan, 1, 27, 28, 51, 70, 77, 80, 93, 123
Chemonucleolysis, 106
Cluneal nerve, 17
Confirmed disc lesion, 27, 28
Correlation between pain area, Spinal nerve, and lesion, 26

Database, 107
   double pain syndromes, 112
   single pain syndromes, 107
   three or more pain syndromes, 113
   totals for all pain syndromes, 115
Dejerine's Triad, 35, 80
Dermatome, 15
Diathermy, 75. *See also* pulsed diathermy, 130
Disc, 9, 28, 80
Disrelation. *See* Relation, 21

Electrotherapy, 102
Electrolyte imbalance, 10
EMG (electroneuromyography) test, foreword, 94
Examination procedures, 35

Fabere test, 38. *See also* Patrick sign, 38
Facet syndrome, 51

Failed spinal surgery, 33
Femoral nerve, 13
Fibrocartilage, 9
Fibrosis, 38
First lumbar nerve, 13
Fixation, 21
Foramen, 10

Gaenslen's test, 55
Gemellus muscle, 19
Genitofemoral nerve, 13
Gluteal muscle, 65, 66
Gluteal pain syndrome, 6, 65

Hip lesion, 38
   crepitus, 63

Iliohypogastric nerve, 12
Ilioinguinal nerve, 12
Impairment rating, 97
Inguinal pain syndrome, 5, 57
Interspinous ligament, 11
Interspinales muscle, 10
Intertranversarii, 10

Joint bind, 21

Kemp sign, 35
Knee lesion, 69, 71, 73, 74

Labia, 58
Lamina, 9
Lateral femoral pain syndrome, 7
Lateral femoral nerve, 7, 73
Lesion (spinal), 21
   classification of a spinal lesion, 22
   definition of a spinal lesion, 22
   primary lesion, 23
      definition of a primary lesion, 23
   reaction,
      anterior primary rami, 25

posterior primary rami, 24
secondary lesion, 23
  definition of a secondary lesion, 23
sub-classification of a spinal lesion, 24
subluxation disrelation lesion, 22
  definition, 22
symptoms of a spinal lesion, 24
  definition of the term "symptom," 24
Leg region, 6
Ligamentum flavum, 9
Linders test, 39
Load limit, 26
Locking, 21
Longissimus thoracis, 10
Longitudinal ligament, 9
Low back region, 3
Lumbar pain syndrome, 5, 51
Lumbar plexus, 12, 31
  femoral nerve, 13
  first lumbar nerve, 12
  genitofemoral nerve, 13
  iliohypogastric nerve, 12
  ilioinguinal nerve, 12
  lateral femoral nerve, 13
  saphenous nerve, 18
  twelfth thoracic nerve, 12
Lymphatics, 38

Manipulation, 102
Massage, 102
Matrix changes, 10
Mechanism of pain, 31
Medication, 105
Meningeal nerve, 12
Meralgia parenthetica, 73
Metamerism, 19, 81
Motion, 9
Motor unit (spinal), 9
  anatomy, 9
    anterior longitudinal ligament, 9
    anterior portion, 9
    disc, 9
    foramenal contents, 10
    injury/reaction, 10, 21, 27
    interspinous ligament, 9
    intervertebral foramen, 10
    ligamentum flavum, 9
    middle portion, 9
    motion, 9
    posterior longitudinal ligament, 9
    posterior portion, 9
    supraspinous ligament, 9
MRI (nuclear magnetic resonance imaging) scan, 1, 27, 28, 51, 77, 93, 123
Multifidus muscle, 10
Muscles,
  interspinales muscle, 10
  intertransversarii, 10
  longissimus thoracis muscle, 10
  multifidus muscle, 10
  psoas, 33
  quadratus lumborum, 11, 27, 33
  rotatories muscle, 10
  semispinalis muscle, 10
Muscles of the back, 10

Negative joint reaction, 2
Nerves,
  anterior femoral nerve, 18
  genitofemoral nerve, 110, 127
  iliohypogastric nerve, 18
  ilioinguinal nerve, 18
  inferior cluneal nerves, 17
  lateral femoral nerve, 19
  ninth, tenth, eleventh thoracic nerves, 10
  paraspinal nerves, 15, 17
  posterior femoral nerve, 19
  saphenous nerve, 18
  sciatic nerve, 19
  superior cluneal nerves, 17
  sural nerve, 19
  twelfth thoracic nerve, 17, 18, 19

Objective symptoms, 125
Obturator muscle, 19

Pain syndromes, 2
  criteria, 4
  identification, 3
  pain mechanism, 32
    anterior femoral syndrome, 6
    gluteal syndrome, 5
    inguinal syndrome, 5
    lateral femoral syndrome, 7
    lumbar syndrome, 5
    paraspinal syndrome, 4
    posterior femoral syndrome, 7
    Thomas syndrome, 6
Paraspinal pain syndrome, 4, 45, 46
Patrick sign, 38. See also Fabere test, 38
Pelvic region, 5
Posterior femoral nerve, 19, 77
Posterior femoral pain syndrome, 7, 77
Posterior primary rami, 12, 17, 31
Postfixed plexus, 17
Prefixed plexus, 17
Primary lesion, 23
Primary subluxation, 23
Protective mechanism, 32
Psoas muscle, 27, 33
Pulsed diathermy, 130

Quadratus lumborum muscle, 11, 27, 33
Quiescent period, 42

Reactive mechanism, 32
Reactive rating (examination), 42
Recurrent sinuvertebral nerve, 12
Relation, 21
Restriction, 21
Rotatores muscle, 10

Sacral nerves, 13
  great sciatic nerve, 13
  posterior femoral nerve, 13
  sural nerve, 13
Sacral plexus, 13
  great sciatic nerve, 13
  posterior femoral nerve, 13
  saphenous nerve, 13
  sural nerve, 13
Sacroiliac lesion, 55
Sacrospinalis. *See* Muscles, 10
Saphenous nerve, 18, 70
Secondary lesion, 23
Secondary subluxation, 23
Segmental examination findings, 42
Segmental testing, 41
Semispinalis muscle, 10
Sicard's test, 35
Side posture treatment, 102
  torsion roll,
    thoracolumbar region, 103
    4th, 5th lumbar, 104
S.L.R. (straight leg raising) test, 36
  sitting, 39
Small sciatic nerve
    (posterior femoral), 19, 78
Soto Hall test, 39
Spinal joint lesion, 21
  classification, 22
  definition, 22
  primary spinal joint lesion, 23
  reaction—anterior primary rami, 24
  reaction—posterior primary rami, 25
  secondary spinal joint lesion, 23
  symptoms of a spinal joint lesion, 24
Spinous process, 9
Sprain,
  definition, 125
Strain,
  definition, 125

Subjective symptoms, 125
Subluxation, 21
  (subluxation/disrelation lesion),
    definition, 22
  sequel, 22, 26
  sub-classification, 24
  symptoms, 26
Supraspinal ligament, 9, 11, 33, 53
Surgical intervention, 106
Symptoms (spinal lesion), 24

Testes, 58
Tests for low back, pelvic and leg pain,
  bowstring sign, 35
  Braggards test, 80
  buckling sign, 35
  Dejerine's Triad, 35
  Fabere (Patrick), 38
  Gaenslen's test, 55
  Kemp sign, 35
  Linders, 39
  percussion test, 35
  Sicard's test, 35
  sitting-straight leg raising, 39
  Soto Hall, 39
  spinal segmental examination, 41
  straight leg raising, 37
  Turyn's test, 35
Thomas pain syndrome, 6, 61
Thoracic nerves, 12, 16
Three-joint complex, 28
  versus diagnosis of spinal joint
    lesions in low back/leg pain, 28
Torsion roll, 103, 104

Ultrasound (ultrasonography) scan, 1, 93, 105
  pulsed ultrasonography, 75

Vertebral testing, 41
  body position, 41
  findings, 42
  testing form #111, 138
  tissue reaction, 42

X-ray (roentgen ray) photographs, 1, 27, 28, 41, 51, 62, 63, 70, 74, 80, 96, 98, 123